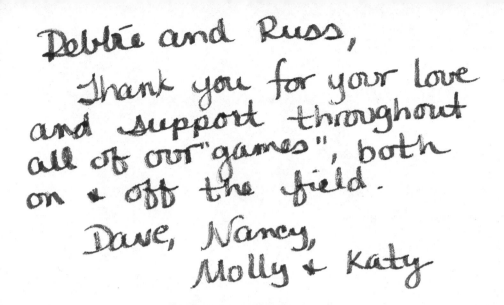

Debbie and Russ,
    Thank you for your love
and support throughout
all of our "games", both
on & off the field.
    Dave, Nancy,
        Molly & Katy

They laugh that win.
— Shakespeare

Debbie & Russ —

Best wishes

Bob Evans

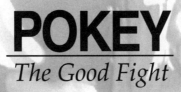

POKEY
The Good Fight

Pokey Allen and Bob Evancho

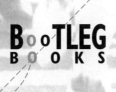

B**oo**TLEG
B **o o** K S

Boise, Idaho

LIBRARY OF CONGRESS CATALOG CARD NUMBER: 97-071515
ISBN: 0-9658911-0-0

Designed by Chris Latter
Front and back cover photographs by Chuck Scheer

To Jennie
— P.A.

To my parents with love and gratitude
And to Mike Brick
—B.E.

Acknowledgements

Ernest Duncan "Pokey" Allen Jr. died of cancer in the early morning hours of Monday, December 30, 1996—30 days short of his 54th birthday—at St. Patrick Hospital in his hometown of Missoula, Montana. His body was cremated later that day.

The idea for this book began in late March 1996 when I interviewed Pokey for an article in *FOCUS*, Boise State University's alumni magazine. As fellow BSU employees, Pokey and I had met briefly on a few occasions, but we barely knew each other. The purpose of the article, I explained at the time, was to provide *FOCUS'* readers with both a first-person account of his battle with cancer, which at the time was in remission, and a medical update.

In the days that followed I found his story to be quite riveting; it was much more interesting and compelling than what could be contained in a single magazine article. Then he began to tell me stories about himself—humorous anecdotes and hilarious misadventures unrelated to his illness or his tenure as BSU's head football coach. That's when the gears started turning.

"You know, your comeback from cancer is a great story in itself," I said. "But you've had an interesting career and an eventful life before that. I think it has the makings of a book." He immediately dismissed such a notion. "Who? Me?" he laughed. "You gotta be kidding! Nobody is interested in my life or what I have to say." I finally convinced him otherwise; I'm glad I did. In a matter of days we agreed to become co-authors and began working on this book. For the next nine months—until two weeks before his death—he shared with me his thoughts and divulged details of his life.

We originally intended to end this book on an upbeat and optimistic note—with Pokey coaching the 1996 Broncos in their inaugural season as a Division I-A team and his cancer in remission. Tragically, the disease that he fought so bravely eventually prevailed.

Pokey was best known as a football coach, but to those who knew and loved him, he was much more. As a public figure, Pokey was involved in a number of charitable efforts, but he never sought the spotlight when helping a worthy cause.

Despite his illness, he remained in good humor while maintaining a steadfast effort to defeat his affliction, and through his two-year ordeal he was never heard to utter, "Why me?" Throughout his life Pokey had a seize-the-day philosophy that was infectious. He will be remembered for his accomplishments as a coach, but he will also be remembered for the way he attacked life—whether it was academics, sports or the illness that finally ended his life.

Pokey was a highly successful and immensely popular college football coach, serious when it mattered, yet with few of the profession's traditional pretensions. In his 10-plus seasons at Boise State and Portland State he compiled an 86-41-2 record. In his seven years at PSU, he led the Vikings to the NCAA Division II playoffs five times and to the national championship game twice. In 1994, his second year at BSU, he guided the Broncos to the second-best turnaround in Division I-AA football history and to the national title game. During those years he won numerous coaching awards. And in the process he gained widespread respect and admiration in the communities where he coached.

Yes, Pokey Allen was a great football coach and gifted leader. But you don't define a man like Pokey in such facile terms. He was many things to many people. In my eyes, he became the epitome of grace and courage in the face of death because the cancer that ended his life never defeated his will.

This book chronicles Pokey's life—his childhood, his adolescence, his playing and coaching careers, his battle with cancer—in his own words. But telling his story was much more than a two-man project; and this book would not have been written without the support and assistance of many people.

During the course of writing this book, several of Pokey's relatives provided invaluable information and perspective on his life. They include his mother Esther Allen; his sister and brother-in-law Jennie and Jack Kirschling; his former wives Barbara Allen Callaghan and Tammy Kettlewell; and his cousin Madeline Pinsoneault.

I am also indebted to many of Pokey's friends and colleagues, all of whom graciously shared their time. From the Missoula County High School Class of '61: John Oblizalo, Larry Schmautz, Dale Schwanke and Tom Stage along with former MCHS teacher Erwin Byrnes. Also David Boyd, Jerry Bradley, Kate Johnson Hart, Cap Hedges, Diane Hemingson, Janie

Hemingway, Jon Miller, Mike Munsey, Sherri Niesen, Ken Staninger, Jeff Taylor, Steve Weaver and Mike Young.

The following men coached with, over, or for Pokey. They all provided important information about his career: Ned Alger, Chris Beaton, Don Bailey, Al Borges, Gene Carlson, George Hughes, Lary Kuharich, Tom Mason, Barry Sacks and Dave Stromswold.

Pokey had an outstanding relationship with the press, which was reflected in the great alacrity with which the following media members assisted in sharing information: Steve Brandon, Paul Buker, Reil Cummins, Michael D'Orso, Terry Frei, Ken Goe, Dana Haynes, Carolyn Holly, George Giese, Art Lawler, Harry Minium, Paul J. Schneider, Steve Wieberg and Jeff Welsch.

A key component in a book of this nature is the assistance of sports information directors. My thanks to the following SIDs who were so generous with their time: Glenn Alford, Idaho State; Paul Allen, Mankato State; Dave Cook, Eastern Washington; Dave Guffey, Montana; James Phillips, Simon Fraser; Kevin Reneau, Cal-Berkeley; Larry Sellers, Portland State; and Bruce Woodbury, Utah. Also, thanks to Jim Dorash, B.C. Lions director of media relations.

Special thanks to Max Corbet, Boise State's senior sports information director.

I am also grateful to Gene Bleymaier, Larry Burke, Dr. Carolyn Collins, Jon Cox, Eldon Edmundson, Mark Freeman, Fred Goode, Roy Love, Dave McNally, Larry Questad and Dr. George Wade for their time and help.

My thanks to those who helped at the technical end: transcribers Roxanne Gunner, Sandy Lee, Suzan Raney and Kathy Schindler; proofreaders Jennifer Benedict, Joe H. Evancho and Ed Morrison; photographers John Kelly and Chuck Scheer; designer Chris Latter; and copy editor Susette Freeman.

Most of all, thanks to my wife, Sue Evancho, a proficient proofreader and an astute business manager—but most important, a totally selfless parent who served as both mom and dad to our three young children during much of this project.

Sadly, Pokey did not live to add his own contributions to these acknowledgements. But I feel honored to have this opportunity to speak for him here.

Bob Evancho
Boise, Idaho
July 1997

Prologue

It was Pokey Allen's custom to spend the holidays in Missoula, Montana; 1996 was to be no exception. But he knew this trip to his hometown would be his last. Allen, the former head football coach at Boise State University, had resigned his position two weeks earlier when it became apparent he was losing his two-year battle with rhabdomyosarcoma—a rare and aggressive tissue cancer.

On December 17 he left Boise, Idaho, for Vancouver, British Columbia, to renew the experimental cancer treatments he had undergone in Canada from the previous August to early November. The alternative medication had slowed the cancer's growth and given him a reprieve; it allowed him to return to Boise State to coach the final two games of the 1996 season. But 17 days after the Broncos' November 23 season finale, a CAT scan revealed the cancer once again was spreading—with a vengeance—forcing his return to Canada.

After spending a week in Vancouver, Allen set out for Missoula. His plane trip was delayed by a severe snowstorm; still, he managed to reach his hometown on December 23. Waiting for him were the most important people in his life—his mother, his sister and her family, his three-year-old daughter, Taylor, and many longtime friends.

Pokey was home.

Then he summoned up his last reserves of strength to fulfill his Christmas Eve tradition. Gaunt and hollow-eyed, the tumor in his chest festering, the cancer in his lungs slowly killing him, Allen somehow managed to make his appointed rounds that night. His visits were brief; he knew he was fading. He met a group of buddies at Stockman's Bar in downtown Missoula. He then went to The Depot, a popular restaurant owned by one of his best friends, Mike Munsey, for dinner. He hardly ate. He raised his glass of wine to his lips a couple of times, but he couldn't drink it. "You know, Munce," he said to his friend as they sat together in front of the restaurant's fireplace, "this will be my last Christmas with Taylor."

He spent Christmas Day with family and friends, his condition rapidly deteriorating. On Thursday, December 26, in a state of severe weakness, he collapsed, breaking his nose, and was admitted to Missoula's St. Patrick Hospital. On Sunday he lapsed into a coma.

NEW YEAR'S DAY 1997 in Missoula was cold, wet, gray. Clouds shrouded the nearby hills. The record snowfall from the previous week gave way to a soft, intermittent drizzle, turning side streets and alleys into rivers of slush. In the middle of the day Pokey Allen's family and friends gathered to say goodbye. Quietly, respectfully, they filled St. Anthony Catholic Church. Music played. The floral arrangements on the altar included one of white and brown chrysanthemums in the shape of a football. When the mourners had all been seated, Allen's immediate family—his mother, Esther Allen of Missoula; his sister, Jennie Kirschling of Bellevue, Washington, and her family; and his former wife, Barbara Allen Callaghan of Missoula—filed in and filled the front pew.

Allen's three-year-old daughter, Taylor Elizabeth, came to the church with her mother. But at the last minute it was decided to have her remain in the vestibule with a relative. Taylor's mother and others anticipated a great deal of weeping during the service and they feared the child might become distressed and confused at the sight of so much sorrow.

Allen's brother-in-law, Jack Kirschling, walked to the lectern and opened the memorial service with a passage from 2 Timothy 4:6-8: "I am already being poured out like a libation," he read. "The time of my dissolution is near. I have fought the good fight, I have finished the race, I have kept the faith. ..."

The eulogies followed. The first speaker was Boise businessman Jon Miller, a Boise State booster who befriended Allen when he took the school's head coaching job four years earlier. "It's been said that most people can count on one hand the people they've known outside their own families who have made a truly lasting imprint on their own lives," he said. "Pokey was such a person for me, and I know for many of you.

"Wherever he lived and coached—Missoula, Portland and Boise being the most recent—he captivated people and made a lasting impression upon the entire community. He was in each place more than a football coach.

"In Boise he gave our community a gift we will never forget. He made football fun. He gave us hope. He made us winners. He gave us pride. He showed his players and the community how to perform in such a way as to exceed one's capabilities. He showed us what strength of character is all about.

"Like all of us, Pokey wasn't perfect. But he was special—very special. He was always positive. He was a winner in every sense of the word. He taught people to never give up. He made life exciting. He had a special charisma which was contagiously inspiring—some called it magic.

"He made people feel good about themselves. He made the highs euphoric and the lows bearable. But most of all he cared for others. He lent his name and support to every fund drive for a worthy cause that asked for help.

"Many said that football was Pokey's life. He did have a passion for football, but people were Pokey's life. He always wanted to be around people, to please them and to be liked and loved by them. He was the most open, caring, real, unpretentious human being I've ever known."

Pausing to compose himself, Miller continued. "Then there is courage. You cannot think of Pokey and not think of courage during both his good health and bad. In everything he did he never gave up. He always fought back, and in the end he never said 'goodbye.'

"In looking back at Pokey's life, we can all take comfort from knowing that he lived a good and rewarding one. He did what he wanted to do. He did it his way. He touched and helped others—many others."

The next speaker was Allen's longtime friend Ken Staninger, a Missoula real estate businessman and sports agent . "When I sat down to work on this eulogy, the memories of Pokey and the laughter often drove me to tears," he said. Then Staninger regaled the gathering with one of his favorite Pokey stories—about the midnight cruise and how Allen's boat ran out of gas, leaving Pokey and his passengers stranded in the middle of Flathead Lake. "Pokey taught us to laugh at our mistakes," Staninger said, "and that's something we all need."

The last speaker was Mike Munsey, who took his place behind the lectern on the church's altar. "Pokey Allen was my friend," Munsey began. "We can all say that because Pokey collected friends. He never judged us. He made us laugh. He made us feel better about ourselves. He always found something to like in everyone. The most important thing to Pokey was how you treated other people. That's how he measured us as people. He also wanted us to have fun. He would use laughter in everything. He'd say, 'Let's play golf, we'll laugh.'"

Munsey paused to collect himself. "You know," he said, "good friends help make you a better person because they make you want to be like them. How could anyone ever have a better friend than Pokey Allen?"

Then he shared a story: "When Pokey got sick I went to see him in

Boise before he went to Seattle for treatment. We played golf, we had a few beers, we laughed. The last day I was there it rained; we couldn't play golf, so we were just sitting around Pokey's house talking. Then out of nowhere he said to me, 'You know, if I don't make it, you have to do me a favor. You have to tell Taylor about me.' I got tears in my eyes and said to him, 'Are you sure you want me to?'" The church filled with laughter.

"He said, 'You're a mean person,' and we laughed," Munsey continued. "But I knew what he meant. He didn't mean that just for me; he meant it for all of us."

Again Munsey paused before he continued. "I will tell her, as we all will," he said. "I'll tell her he was an 'A' student in high school and a merit scholar. How he was an academic All-American in college.

"I'll tell her about how as a youngster he carried a dictionary with him all the time so he could learn new words and no one could use a word he didn't understand. I'll tell her he went to Boys' State.

"I'll tell her what a great athlete he was—every sport, every position. About how he was an All-American in every sense of the word. I'll also tell her that I think he liked golf best of all.

"I'll tell her about the summer when he was 16 and he and friends Tom Stage and Larry Schmautz and a bunch of guys got jobs on the railroad and how everybody quit but Pokey.

"I'll tell her what he said to me in the hospital just before he died. He said, 'You know, Munce, I'm not a quitter. You tell everyone I never quit. You tell them I never gave up.' Well, he didn't give up. He fought to the very end. Pokey Allen never gave up on himself, and he never gave up on any of us. Ever."

People wept openly as Munsey continued. "I'll tell Taylor how people would come up to Pokey and talk to him like they'd known him forever. And then they'd leave and I'd say, 'Who was that?' and he'd say, 'I have no idea.' He had time for all of us.

"I'll tell her he was the most fun, loving, decent person I ever met. I'll tell her we all loved him. I'll tell her everything I can about Pokey; we all will. But mostly, I'll tell her how much he loved her."

The service ended moments later. Pokey Allen's family and friends slowly filed out. Many were still crying. They shared hugs and tears in the back of the church. Shortly thereafter, many of the mourners gathered at Munsey's restaurant to eat, drink and watch what remained of the New Year's Day bowl games.

That's the way Pokey would have wanted it.

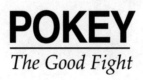

POKEY
The Good Fight

Chapter 1

Why Not *Me?*

I knew something was wrong with my arm, but I still wasn't prepared for the news I was about to receive. I remember walking into the Idaho Sports Medicine Institute, which adjoins our football offices and other athletic department facilities in the Varsity Center on the Boise State campus, feeling a little apprehensive. It was around 2 in the afternoon, Monday, December 19, 1994—six weeks short of my 52nd birthday. George Wade, our team physician, called that morning and said he wanted to see me.

My frame of mind was just fine even though our team had lost the Division I-AA national championship game two days earlier. Physically, it was another story. I had been feeling tired and listless for a few months, and I was hurting from what I thought was a large cyst in my right triceps. A week earlier, Dr. Wade had examined the lump in my upper arm and had me undergo an MRI (magnetic resonance imaging, a computerized X-ray that uses magnetism to capture its images). Two days later, on the morning our team left for Huntington, West Virginia, to play in the title game, he drained the lump and took a biopsy (the removal of tissue for examination). My weary body and ailing arm were bothersome, but no cause for major concern at the time, certainly nothing that would keep me from work or my usual public appearances as BSU's head football coach. In fact, I had just finished speaking to a packed house in the BSU Student Union during the weekly luncheon hosted by the university's booster club. Despite our loss in the national title game the previous Saturday to Youngstown State, the luncheon was upbeat and festive. After all, the '94 Broncos had just completed a remarkable season and we were feeling pretty good about ourselves.

But the laughter and frivolity of the luncheon faded from my mind the minute I saw the troubled look on Wade's face. He led me to one of the examining rooms and closed the door behind him. I don't recall the exact details of that moment, but I *do* remember Wade's words: "Pokey," he said, "you've got cancer."

That was it. No dramatics. No outpouring of emotion, no sudden sick feeling in the pit of my stomach. I wasn't scared, but I must admit I *was* caught off guard. Sure, I knew something was wrong, but *cancer*? My initial reaction? "Oh shit," I think I said.

It was devastating news to say the least. But I also found the whole thing to be somewhat ironic. I mean, I had enjoyed nearly perfect health my entire life. Sure, I had the usual childhood diseases like the mumps, and I remember missing a basketball road trip my sophomore year in high school because of a bad case of the flu. But that was the extent of it. In fact, in all my years of playing sports, I had never been hospitalized overnight, which was pretty amazing when you consider that I incurred my share of injuries.

My meeting with Wade was brief. He went on to explain that I had a rare form of tissue cancer called rhabdomyosarcoma in my right triceps. Unfortunately, the bad news got even worse: This particular cancer, he informed me, is among the most deadly. "OK," I said to Wade. "We obviously have a problem; let's see if there's a solution." A "problem" is putting it mildly. What was to follow would be a fight for my life—a battle I almost lost twice in the ensuing months.

Wade seemed more distressed than I was. But then, he had carried a heavy burden for the past week: He alone knew about my condition. Sure, he wasn't positive it was cancer, but he had a pretty good hunch before we left for Huntington. (I *thought* he seemed overly concerned about my arm during the trip.) But he couldn't be absolutely certain until he got the biopsy results following our return to Boise. And because he didn't want to overburden me as our team prepared to play for the national title, he decided not to say anything. Now it seemed he was second-guessing himself. Should he have told me right away?

Hard to say, but I do know this: George Wade, who has been Boise State's team doctor for 18 years, is a great man. He's compassionate, he cares. I really think the world of him. Was I upset he didn't tell me? Shoot no! I knew there was something wrong when he needed to do a biopsy. For some reason, I just never thought cancer was among the possibilities. So, I asked Wade, where would I have to go to fight this disease? I envisioned innumerable trips to Seattle or Salt Lake City. As it turned out, I only had to drive across town to begin with. "There's a doctor at St. Al's named Carolyn Collins," Wade said. "She specializes in the kind of cancer you have. I'm going to send you right over there to see her."

A couple of hours later, I met Dr. Collins at the St. Alphonsus Cancer Treatment Center. She was very honest and straightforward—blunt even—with her prognosis. "Rhabdomyosarcoma is a child's cancer. It's rare even among children, and it's almost unheard of with people your age," she told me. "But you've got it, and it's a nasty form of cancer. We don't know for certain, but right now you probably have a 40 to 60 percent chance of living through the next three years."

I WAS HOPING that any minute someone would wake me from this nightmare. Unfortunately, it was no dream, and two days later I entered St. Al's to begin the treatment to combat the malignancy in my arm. At least I had one thing going for me: Collins agreed to be my doctor. One of the first things I asked Collins was if I would have to quit coaching. "It depends on how the chemotherapy affects you," she said. "If you handle the chemo OK and adhere to some restrictions, you can probably keep working." And that's exactly what I planned to do.

Two days later, on December 21, the BSU athletic department called a press conference at St. Al's to inform the public of my illness. In a mere 48 hours my life had changed. It seemed I had somehow transformed from this healthy, vigorous football coach into a man whose long-term chance of survival was in serious doubt. All of a sudden I had to tell the world about this disease I could barely pronounce. *Rhabdomyosarcoma*!? It sure sounded ominous, and according to Collins, it was.

"This is an aggressive malignancy," she stated at the press conference. "I think that if you are playing the odds here, the odds that Pokey will be alive ... at age 75 [are] somewhere between 50 and 60 percent." Still, I tried to remain upbeat about my situation. Heck, my chances of surviving had improved by 10 percent over the odds Collins gave me two days earlier. "Shoot," I joked, "I didn't think I had those odds from the first." When Collins mentioned the rarity of the disease (of the less than 1,000 cases diagnosed annually in the U.S. fewer than 10 percent afflict people over 50), I responded with another quip. "This is just super," I said to the reporters who were crammed into the hospital conference room. "I can't even get a normal cancer." When asked about the chemotherapy that loomed ahead, I shrugged and said: "You can drink beer with it. I mean, how bad can it be?"

Given the gravity of the situation, some people thought the blasé attitude and gallows humor I displayed in front of the TV cameras were some kind of denial mechanism. As a matter of fact, I can remember Collins saying, "You're in denial, aren't you?" I said, "No, I'm not in denial. I know what I've got. I know what the odds are. I know exactly what you are telling me. But I'm not going to change; I can handle this. We'll just see what happens. Just tell me what I need to do. Hey, I'm a coach, I'm coachable." I simply wanted to stress to Collins and everyone else that this illness, no matter how serious or life-threatening, was not going to suddenly change my personality. I mean, there are a lot of people who are a lot worse off than me. Basically, I've had a great life, and no matter what was in store, I wasn't going to go down like a whimpering little whiner.

In these kinds of situations, I think most people ask, Why me? But that has never been my style. And that was the point I tried to make at the press conference. "Why *not* me?" I said to the reporters. "It's just a deal that I've got to fight, and we'll see what happens. There's a lot more important things to do than worry about Pokey Allen. There are some children who probably have the same disease. Let's just stud up and get going. I don't want anybody coming up and asking me how I feel. Just say hello. In the whole scheme of the world, this is very small." I wasn't being macho or dramatic—I was being me.

Nevertheless, reality set in immediately following the press conference: I was led away to a treatment room where I underwent a three-hour chemotherapy session in which a dose of two drugs, cyclophosphamide and vincristine, were infused into my body. That was followed by a surgical procedure to implant an intravenous access device called a portacath in my chest. The device was hooked up to a type of fanny pack that contained an outpatient infusion pump which slowly fed yet another chemotherapy drug called adriamycin into my veins. It was necessary to gradually introduce the drug into my system because of its toxicity.

And this was just the beginning. Days, weeks and months of intensive treatment lay ahead. More MRIs, more chemotherapy, surgery to remove the tumor, radiation treatment, a stem-cell transplant and more—lots more.

There was no question about it: I was in big trouble.

Chapter 2

Growing Up

I must admit, my illness was a shocker—in no small part because I'm unaware of any history of cancer in my family. In fact, my mom is in her late 70s and still in relatively good health. My dad died in 1971 at the age of 70 of complications stemming from polycystic kidney disease, diabetes and heart failure.

My dad was a 23-year veteran of the Montana Highway Patrol and a popular figure in Missoula, Montana, during the more than 25 years he lived there. He never discussed his childhood, but I have a feeling it was pretty unhappy. When he was around 15 or 16 years old, he lied about his age, enlisted in the Marine Corps during World War I and fought in Europe, where he was wounded. He rejoined the Marines during World War II despite the fact he was already in his 40s. He never told me how he was injured. But I can remember as a kid when we went to the beach or the lake, I could see some scars on his body that I think were war wounds. I'm not sure if he was shot or hit by a grenade or injured some other way. He never discussed it—at least not with me.

He was a large, barrel-chested man, 6-foot-3, 230 pounds. He played high school football in Great Falls, Montana, and then college ball at Montana Wesleyan, now called Rocky Mountain College, in Billings. He met my mom, the former Esther Johnson, in Superior, Montana, in 1941; he was 41 and she was 23 when they got married on April 15, 1942. They didn't waste any time starting a family; I was born on January 29, 1943, in Superior. As a football player, my dad was a big, lumbering lineman; that's how he got the nickname "Pokey." When I came along, I was named Ernest Duncan Allen Jr. and inherited the nickname "Little Pokey." As I got older the "Little" eventually faded from my nickname, thank goodness. On August 2, 1944, my only sibling, Jennie Lee, was born. That same summer my dad was transferred from Superior to the Highway Patrol post in

Missoula, a move of about 60 miles down Interstate 90. On September 1, 1944, he began his new assignment, and around the same time we moved into a small house in Missoula.

My childhood was pretty typical for a kid growing up in Montana. With 11 cousins living in Superior, my sister and I weren't lacking for childhood companions. Interestingly, all 11 of my cousins were from one family, the Doyles. Like most kids, summer was my favorite time of year. With my dad often working odd hours, my mom, my sister and I spent a good portion of our summers in Superior with the Doyles. My aunt was my mom's sister and my uncle was the town doctor, the only one in Superior; he delivered both Jennie and me. While the Doyles were devout Catholics (they must have been with 11 kids), our family took a less dogmatic approach to religion. My dad was kind of an atheist and my mother was a Lutheran. As kids, Jennie and I would go to the local Lutheran church with our mom most Sundays. Pretty soon it was just my mother and Jennie; basically I wasn't interested in religion until I got to college. Then I briefly became a First Baptist. My religious beliefs today? I have moral convictions, and I believe strongly in treating other people as I would want to be treated. I believe in God, but I'm just not sure that I necessarily believe in religion.

As you might imagine, a house filled with 13 kids made for some pretty crazy times during those summers in Superior. Being with my sister and my cousins was great fun. It was an idyllic time for me. We spent those days playing in the hills and mountains near my cousins' home; my older cousins set traps and we'd catch coyote, fox and beaver. My cousin David and I were especially close. We were born the same year and were in the same grade; he was the closest thing I had to a brother. On many summer mornings David and I would leave his house at dawn, hike up to nearby Flat Creek and fish most of the day. It was a great way to be a kid. But when I turned eight, organized baseball took over as the focal point of my summers, and I didn't go to Superior as often. The next 10 or so summers were dominated by baseball as I progressed from Little League to Babe Ruth League to American Legion. Part of the reason that I enjoyed the game so much was because I was pretty good.

Luckily, baseball isn't a real expensive sport to play. I say that because when I think about my childhood, I now realize our financial situation wasn't the greatest. Our first house in Missoula was tiny with just one bedroom, and my dad's patrol car doubled as our family car. In 1950, when I was in the first grade, we moved into a modest three-bedroom house on the west side of Missoula, which wasn't a slum but was definitely the poor side of town. Our new home cost $6,000, which my dad thought was an outrageous price. My dad's salary was basically our only source of income, and at times it seemed like my parents lived paycheck to paycheck, squeezing my dad's earnings to cover our needs as best they could. My mom occasionally worked a part-time job at a local newsstand, but it didn't pay much. I don't know how much my dad was making while my sister and I were growing up, but when I signed a pro football contract in 1965 for $10,500 he told me it was more than his annual salary.

But as a youngster I never felt deprived, never felt poor or ashamed. Despite our modest existence, my parents were wonderful providers whose top priority always was the well-being of their children. With the exception of cigarettes, I rarely recall my parents buying anything for themselves. Both my parents smoked a lot, but they rarely drank. In fact, I really can't remember seeing them drink after I turned nine or so. We weren't the kind of family where the parents would have a martini before dinner or a bottle of wine with our meal; it was too expensive for one thing. The one "extravagant" purchase my folks made during my childhood was when they saved enough money to buy our first TV in the mid-1950s, which most American families were doing at that time. One show we watched regularly was *Highway Patrol* starring Broderick Crawford. My dad said he hated the show because it wasn't realistic, but he'd watch it anyway because there wasn't a lot to choose from back then.

For me, television was merely a diversion; as a youngster and a teenager most of my time was occupied playing sports. Our house was a block from Missoula's Lowell School, which had a large playfield that provided my friends and me with a year-round sports venue. Until the ninth grade, youth baseball and fifth- through eighth-grade basketball were the only organized sports available for kids in Missoula. But from grades one through eight I would play pickup football and basketball games almost every day during those seasons. I can remember playing football as a 10-year-old with a bunch of older kids and catching my first pass; I was extremely excited even though it was just a neighborhood game on a school playground. To me, it was like being a star wide receiver in a real game. During the winter months when my friends and I couldn't get into Lowell's gym, we would shovel any snow that was on the outdoor basketball courts and play pickup games, no matter how cold it was—and it can get mighty cold in Missoula during certain times of the year. But we didn't think anything of it. I thought it was a great environment for my sister and me to grow up in.

Once I started playing baseball, football and basketball, I lost what little interest I had in hunting and fishing. My dad taught me how to shoot a .22-caliber rifle, and I can vaguely remember hunting for jackrabbits, but I didn't enjoy it. Fortunately, my dad wasn't much of a hunter either. Even though he was a cop, my dad didn't like guns and didn't want them around the house. As an adult I once went duck hunting with a friend; all I recall is being cold, wet and miserable and taking a shot at a duck and hoping I wouldn't hit it. And the last time I can remember going fishing was when I was about 15. Our next-door neighbor wanted to take me fishing, so I went. I haven't fished since. I find it extremely boring.

MY DAD WAS nothing if not demanding. As a cop and an ex-Marine his demeanor could be gruff and authoritarian. When Jennie and I were very young he was a typical doting father who adored his children and was not afraid to outwardly show his affection for us. But as we got older, the almost unavoidable conflicts between offspring and parent manifested themselves in our household at times. He hit me only once; after that he never needed to. One day when I was about 15 I was late for lunch. When my mom asked me where I had been, I made some smart-ass remark. Well, my dad happened to be standing there. First of all, he wouldn't tolerate my sister or me being late for anything, and when I sassed my mom … well, he backhanded me. To this day, I'm rarely late for anything. My dad and sister were both quite hardheaded, which led to occasional clashes. In my case, our source of friction was my athletic pursuits. My dad wanted perfect kids and was quick to criticize my sister and me when his expectations weren't met. For the most part, my sister and I got along great with our dad, and I know he always had our best interests at heart. Still, he could be difficult to live with at times.

My dad gave me plenty of support during my days in youth and high school sports—too much sometimes. I guess you could say he pushed me. In fact, his meddling got so bad that my mom eventually wouldn't allow him to attend my games. I remember one Little League game when I faced this really good pitcher named Tom Boone for the first time. Boone, who went to Harvard and is now an attorney in Missoula, was a great athlete and about three years older than me. When you have a nine-year-old batter going up against a hard-throwing 12-year-old pitcher, it's usually a mismatch. My situation was no different; I never took the bat off my shoulder and Boone struck me out on three pitches. Well, my dad, who was in the stands, came out on the field and started hollering at me and telling me that I had to swing the bat; it was hardly what you would call constructive criticism. I mean, he was mad! In another game I dropped a fly ball and he started yelling at me again. His tirades were frequent, and it got to be pretty unnerving and embarrassing; eventually my mom banned him from all of my athletic contests.

My dad pretty much ruled the roost, but this was one time my mom put her foot down. After that, he rarely went to any of my games. Later, when I was playing football in high school, I could see his patrol car parked outside the field, but he would never come in the stadium and sit in the bleachers. And occasionally he would attend a basketball game. But he couldn't handle it. He'd start yelling at me right in the middle of the game, and the argument would often continue that night at home. As much as I loved sports, it wasn't much fun when he acted that way.

I think there were four primary reasons why my dad could be so irascible at times. First, I think he was like a lot of fathers who are former athletes and want to vicariously relive their athletic success through their sons. You know, I think he probably felt frustrated. I'm told he was a really good football player in college and high school, but back then scholarships were rare and he had to work for everything he got. Second, I think he had serious money problems. Born in 1900, my dad, like millions of others his age, never fully recovered from the financial ravages of the Depression; it was evident that he and my mom almost always struggled to make ends meet. Third was his job. I mean, not only was being a policeman in Montana in the '50s unprofitable, being a cop anywhere anytime is stressful. Fourth was the generation gap that existed between my dad and my sister and me. After all, by the time Jennie and I were in high school he was pushing 60 and not in the greatest health; it was apparent he had trouble relating to us, and vice versa. When I consider all these factors, I think I have a better understanding of why he was the way he was.

According to my cousin, Madeline Pinsoneault, my father was "a good dad, but a very strict dad." I think she had a pretty good perspective on the dynamics at work among the members of our family. The fourth-oldest child of the Doyle family, Madeline lived with us her freshman and sophomore years (the academic years I was in grades five and six) while she attended Sacred Heart Academy, the Catholic high school in Missoula. "I think Butch [my family's nickname for me] didn't like to rock the boat and basically did what his dad wanted," she said. "Jennie, on the other hand, was more like her dad—headstrong, which at times led to clashes between those two. I think my uncle could be intimidating because of his size. It was obvious he loved his kids, but at the same time when he said something he meant it, and at times it was best to walk softly around him."

None of this is meant to say there weren't good times. I can recall my dad spending a great deal of time teaching my buddies and me how to play baseball when we were kids. I remember lots of summer nights when he'd pitch to us for hours, throwing hundreds of pitches—and he was usually the only parent out there with us. He was a tough dad, but he and my mom did everything in their power to provide Jennie and me with the comforts and necessities of a healthy, normal upbringing. With the exception of our arguments about my athletic performances, we usually got along just fine. And there were plenty of times when he'd show his compassionate side. For instance, it seemed he couldn't stand the thought of me being cooped up in my room when I was grounded. I can remember more than once when I'd be sitting in my room serving my "sentence," and he would walk in and say, "You know, you're supposed to be grounded, but I can't do that. Ah, shoot … get outta here, go join your friends."

When I think about it now, my dad's style of parenting seemed somewhat paradoxical. Perhaps Jennie put it best. "His love was unconditional," she said years later. "Problem was, he was very controlling, and I think maybe he loved us so much that sometimes it was hard for us to develop our own identity." Several years after my dad died Larry Schmautz, one of my best friends in high school, made an interesting observation. "When Pokey's dad would talk about his son's athletic accomplishments there would be this gleam in his eye," Larry recalled. "It was obvious Pokey's dad was very proud of his son; what I think he feared was Pokey getting a big head over all the attention he was receiving as a star athlete. I think if Pokey ever started to get a big head, his dad put him in his place. In doing so I think his dad helped develop in Pokey a trait he has always had—humility."

I think part of the reason I excelled in sports and academics early on was because I was afraid of my dad. Jennie, on the other hand, had different priorities—despite our father's threats. My dad used to bitch at Jennie all the time for not doing better in school. In grade school and high school I was by far the better student. It wasn't that she was a poor student; on the contrary, she was very bright. It just seemed she was more interested in having fun than seriously pursuing academics. (As a student at the University of Montana she took her studies a bit more seriously and has gone on to enjoy a successful career as an insurance executive.)

Nevertheless, the fact I was a better student really pissed her off when we were kids. And I used to rub it in whenever I could. It was a long time ago, but I remember one episode when I got her in trouble. When I was in the fourth grade and Jennie was in the third, Lowell School combined the top students in those two grades into one class. During one portion of a lesson when we were supposed to be studying, I noticed that Jennie was talking (which she did a lot) or doing something wrong; I don't remember exactly what. Anyway, I thought it was my duty to report her to the teacher, so I did. She got caught, and boy was she sore at me! And just to make her madder, I grabbed the classroom dictionary and started reading it—just to show her how a fine, upstanding student *should* behave in class. Actually, I was always trying to excel in academics. Whenever I had the opportunity, I would take a dictionary or a volume from our classroom's encyclopedia and start reading it.

Academics were important, but from my dad's perspective, my athletic career took top priority. He told me as long as I was playing sports I didn't have to work. Although he never said so, I like to think he made that promise because he saw my athletic prowess as my ticket to college. I liked that arrangement, but it was a mixed blessing, for while I was able to concentrate on athletics, I had little or no money throughout high school. Fortunately, our family's basic needs were always met despite our financial hardships. I mean, I didn't exactly have what you would call an elaborate wardrobe as a kid, but I didn't really notice it.

By and large, my childhood years were uneventful and free of tragedy, with one sad exception: My cousin David died in a traffic accident in 1954. When he was 10 David was riding his bicycle on Main Street in Superior when he inexplicably veered in front of a truck and was killed instantly. I still remember when we got the news. I had just watched a movie in a downtown Missoula theater with my mom, Jennie, Madeline and another of David's sisters, Theresa, who was also living with us while attending Sacred Heart Academy. As we were leaving the theater my dad pulled up in his squad car and told us David had been killed. It was a sorrowful scene, to say the least. My mom and sister and two cousins started bawling right there on the sidewalk, and my dad and I didn't know what to do. Like I said, at one time David was the closest thing I had to a brother. But by the time of the accident, I wasn't spending much time in Superior and we were no longer inseparable like we had been. Nevertheless, it was one of the saddest moments in my life.

Chapter 3

All-Around Athlete

For some reason, I was always a jittery kid, especially when I was playing sports. It wasn't so much that I lacked self-confidence, but I just felt nervous and ill at ease in the spotlight. Nonetheless, my baseball career, especially my pitching, continued to flourish as I entered my teens, and during the summer of 1957, my final season in Missoula's Babe Ruth League, I had what I suppose you could call a banner year. At least that's what it says in the newspaper clippings from my mom's scrapbook.

As a 14-year-old pitcher and outfielder for the KXLL Knights, my batting average was better than .400 and my win-loss record was around 9-2 with six shutouts. Those shutouts included a pair of no-hitters and a one-hitter in which I struck out 18 of 21 batters I faced. Still, my Babe Ruth coaches, John Campbell and Harry Helman, felt I could have been even better if I hadn't been such a bundle of nerves. In a scouting report they described me as a "worrier." As for my potential as an American Legion player, they wrote, "Brought along slowly, he can develop into a splendid pitcher. [He was] easily one of the best in the Babe Ruth League last year. A clean-cut youngster, Allen can grow and learn fast."

I don't mean to brag, but I might have been the most highly touted athlete among Montana's crop of incoming high school freshmen in the fall of 1957. In addition to being one of the top players in Missoula's Babe Ruth League, I also enjoyed an outstanding basketball career at Lowell School. During the two years that I played on the team that combined Lowell's seventh and eighth graders, our records were 7-2 and 10-1, respectively. In fact, Tom Stage and Larry Schmautz, rivals from Willard School who became teammates and two of my best friends in high school, told me I was one of the best and most competitive basketball and baseball opponents they had ever met. When I left Lowell, I was 5-foot-11, 152 pounds, and I could run as fast and throw a baseball as hard as anyone my age. Unfortunately, my speed—both running and throwing—didn't improve all that much and I grew only two more inches during the next four years.

I wasn't a wallflower when I entered Missoula County High School, but at the same time I certainly didn't consider myself a leader—at least not in a boisterous and conspicuous sense. Back then, I thought an effective leader did so with few words and many deeds. (After nearly 30 years of coaching at the college and pro level, I've had to modify that philosophy and become more vocal at times, but I still believe actions have more power than words.) Despite the fact I was a good student and a standout athlete, I guess I was just a bashful kid as a high school freshman. You'd think I would eventually learn to relax, but I never really did until I went away to college. Sure, most teenagers feel socially awkward and self-conscious at one time or another, but for me such anxiety seemed constant. And talk about stage fright! I was petrified at the thought of public speaking, which many people find pretty ironic today.

In spite of my shyness, I was actually elected class president my freshman year (I ran because the girl I was dating wanted me to), but I never felt comfortable in a leadership role until several years later. As class president my basic duties were to start the meeting of class officers and lead the pledge of allegiance. But doing something as simple as that made me nervous as hell and sometimes I would feel sick to my stomach just thinking about it. What made me so uptight and nervous throughout my teenage years? I'm not really sure. I think part of it was because I was the type who had to please everyone, especially my dad, which was darn near impossible.

I THINK I might have been able to perform at a higher level as a high school athlete if I hadn't been so tense all the time, but I still managed to have a highly successful career highlighted by two state basketball championships. My four years at Missoula County High were consumed by sports—football in the fall, basketball in the winter, track in the spring and American Legion baseball in the summer. Basketball was my favorite sport, baseball was my best, track my worst and football somewhere in between. When I competed for the Missoula Spartans in the late 1950s and early '60s, we were in Montana's only Class AA division, the state's largest classification. Our league was called the Big 10—Livingston, Kalispell, Anaconda, Great Falls, Billings Senior, Butte Central, Butte Public, Helena,

Bozeman—those were our rivals.

Interestingly, three of the top performers in Montana high school sports history—Wayne Estes of Anaconda, Larry Questad of Livingston and Dave McNally of Billings—played at the same time I did. And those three weren't just good; they went on to become world-class athletes—Estes in basketball, Questad in track and McNally in baseball. As an all-around high school athlete, I think I held my own with them, but they clearly were unparalleled in their top sports during the years we competed against one another. McNally graduated from Billings Central in 1960 while Estes, Questad and I graduated in '61, so our paths crossed regularly on the diamond, the track, the gridiron and the basketball court.

Estes wasn't just a good basketball player, he was projected as a first-round pick in the 1965 NBA draft before his untimely death. After a remarkable career at Anaconda he went on to play at Utah State, where he was a consensus All-American and the nation's second-leading scorer, behind Rick Barry of Miami, his senior year. As a junior he was named Player of the Year by *Coach & Athletes Magazine* after averaging 28 points and 13 rebounds a game for the Aggies during the 1963-64 season. An all-star lineman on Anaconda's football team and one of the state's top shot-putters, Estes was one of the best high school basketball players in state history—if not *the* best. When comparisons with Estes are made, the player mentioned most often is Mike Lewis, a 6-7 center who starred for Missoula after I graduated and went on to play college ball for Duke and in the ABA. Who was the best? I'm not sure; those two were in a class by themselves. I speak from firsthand experience because I not only played against Estes in high school, but I also competed against Lewis in a couple of alumni basketball games.

Tragically, Estes was killed in a freak accident on the evening of February 8, 1965, less than two hours after he had set a Nelson Field House single-game scoring mark with 48 points against the University of Denver to go over the 2,000-point mark in his career. Following the game he and a companion were driving home when they came upon a car wreck not too far from the USU campus. In the darkness, the 6-6 Estes apparently didn't see a live electrical wire dangling from a power pole damaged in the crash. As he and his companion approached the wreck, his head brushed against the wire and he was electrocuted; his shorter companion was not hurt.

Questad, who attended Livingston's Park County High, was one of the fastest runners I have ever seen in my life and arguably the greatest sprinter in the history of Montana high school track and field. In fact, Questad, who is now a Boise businessman, was on the 1968 U.S. Olympic track team and finished sixth in the 200-meter dash in Mexico City—the event that became a cause célèbre after U.S. medal winners Tommie Smith and John Carlos raised black-gloved fists during the national anthem.

I was no slowpoke, but when I ran against Questad in the 100-yard dash, he was usually 10 yards ahead of me after my first two steps. Of course, when you're running the 100 in 9.6 seconds and the 220 in 21 flat, you're not going to have much competition—especially in Montana. He was virtually unbeatable in the 100, the 220 and the low hurdles. He also used his blazing speed to play basketball, baseball and football for Livingston. Questad earned an academic scholarship to Stanford after he graduated from high school and enjoyed a stellar college career as a sprinter before making the '68 Olympic team. Thirty-five years have passed since Questad graduated from Livingston, and many of his records still stand.

Needless to say, my track career was nothing like Questad's, but I considered myself a valuable member of Missoula's team because of my versatility; with the possible exception of the long jump I didn't really excel in any single event. In dual meets I would usually finish around third in the 100 and 220 and second in the 440 and low hurdles. From a personal standpoint I didn't really like dual meets because I'd compete in several events and never win anything because I was spread so thin. I enjoyed the state meet, however, because it was two days long and I had time to rest between events. For that reason, I thought I had a shot at both the state championship and the state record in the long jump (22 feet, 8 inches at the time) my senior year. But the injury bug that had plagued me all year long got me again during the long jump competition at the state meet. A knee injury that all but ended my high school football career and put a severe crimp in my senior basketball season was finally starting to heal, but then I reinjured an ankle, also made weak by a football injury, on my first attempt. To add to my frustration, that jump measured 21-10, my best ever at the state meet. So there I was, primed, jumping well—and suddenly hurt again. With my injured ankle, I couldn't improve on my initial jump and had to settle for third place.

LIKE QUESTAD IN track and Estes in basketball, McNally was the dominant American Legion player in Montana at the time—hands down. And like the other two, you could make a strong argument that he was the state's best baseball player ever. He certainly is the most famous: He pitched for 14 years in the majors, posted four consecutive 20-win seasons (1968-71) with the Baltimore Orioles, led the American League in wins with 24 in 1970, and appeared in four World Series. Batting against McNally in Legion ball was the only time I was ever afraid of my opponent during my high school career. I was a good pitcher and a talented everyday player in my own right. In fact, I was scouted by the Los Angeles Dodgers and Kansas City Athletics for a while. But when I faced McNally, I knew I couldn't play pro baseball. I mean, his control wasn't great during those days—he'd average eight to 10 walks per game—but it was scary how fast he was. McNally, who now owns a couple of car dealerships in Billings, was also an outstanding high school basketball player, but his school, Billings Central, was in the Class A division, so our schools didn't play each other.

McNally's Billings Royals were the dominant team in the state during the four years I played Legion ball (Montana doesn't offer interscholastic baseball). And in 1958, my first season on Missoula's Legion club, Billings' pitching staff was awesome. Not only did the Royals, three-time defending state champs at the time, have McNally, they boasted two other outstanding hurlers in John Hooson and Jerry Walters. Our pitching corps, however, was also outstanding—and maybe a little bit deeper than Billings'. Tom Boone, my Little League nemesis, was the ace of our staff, which was bolstered by Mike Dishman, Tim Aldrich, Dale Huber and me. (I started in the outfield, hitting .282 that year, when I didn't pitch.) And despite the Royals' reputation (they had captured seven of the previous eight state titles), we thought we had a chance to beat them in the '58 state playoffs in Helena. Under manager Gene Thompson, who would also be Missoula's head football coach my senior year, we won the state's Western Division title with a 26-10 regular-season record. In fact, I hurled a three-hitter against Billings, outdueling Hooson and McNally, for a 4-2 regular-season victory earlier that summer. My other personal pitching highlight that year was a one-hitter in a 22-0 win over Moscow, Idaho.

In our opening game of the double-elimination state tournament, Aldrich and Huber combined to beat Roundup 5-3. Meanwhile, Billings, the Eastern Division champ, downed Helena 9-2 as Walters struck out 16 and gave up just two hits to the host team. In the second round we surprised Billings 5-0 as Boone threw a four-hitter and struck out 10 Royals. I had a single and a stolen base as we collected seven hits off Hooson. Suddenly we were one win away from taking the state title, which Billings all but considered its personal property. Unfortunately, we couldn't get the job done. In a loser-out game, Billings routed Helena again, this time 8-1, setting up a rematch with our club for the state championship. A win would give us the state crown; a defeat would give both teams one loss each and force a final game the next day. Well, we didn't come close. With his team facing elimination, McNally shut down our batters, striking out 19 and giving up just three hits en route to a 5-0 win. Dishman actually pitched well, holding the Royals hitless through the first five innings. But two singles, three walks, an error and a wild pitch accounted for all five of their runs in the bottom of the sixth.

And if McNally's performance wasn't overpowering enough, Walters came within two outs of a no-hitter the next day in the deciding game as the Royals beat us 2-0 to capture their fourth straight state title. Led by McNally, Billings went on to win the regional playoffs and earned a berth in the American Legion World Series that year. (The Royals also went to the Legion Series and finished second nationally in 1960.) We never really came close to beating Billings in the state playoffs again.

HIGH SCHOOL SPORTS were great fun. But I think I could have been a better player if I had been a little more relaxed. I was always nervous, always pushing myself, always afraid of failure. Nevertheless, it was great being a star athlete in Montana. I mean, high school sports are *the* No. 1 pastime for most small towns across America. In rural states like Montana and Idaho, there's nothing quite like the electricity in the air on a Friday night in the fall during a high school football game. And unlike big cities with many other diversions, the fortunes of the local high school team are of interest to just about everyone in a town like Missoula. Because of that, the local press coverage is usually quite extensive; Missoula was no different. In my mom's scrapbook, there are numerous newspaper clippings with headlines such as "Allen pitches shutout against Billings" and "Allen scores winning touchdown." Sometimes we were made out to be heroes—even if we didn't always deserve the adulation.

Case in point: On September 30, 1960, I suffered a knee injury in the fourth football game of my senior year against Billings Senior and wasn't expected to play the rest of the season. But late in our final game of the year against Flathead High of Kalispell, our starting quarterback, Gary Minster, got hurt and his backup was also unable to play. With the score tied 6-6 it appeared Kalispell, which needed a win to stay in the running for the state championship, was going to do just that as it drove deep into our territory in the closing moments of the game. But the Braves' drive stalled at our seven-yard line and coach Gene Thompson put me in at quarterback with 25 seconds remaining. I took the snap and threw a long pass near midfield, which fell incomplete and stopped the clock with about 10 seconds to go. On the next play I faded back into our own end zone and tossed a weak pass—a wounded duck in football vernacular—in the flat to Dick Campbell, our star halfback. Somehow, Campbell made a difficult catch at the 12-yard line, regained his balance, picked up a couple of blocks near midfield and raced through Kalispell's stunned secondary for the winning score. It was a really lame pass, a floater that totaled all of five yards, completed and turned into a spectacular, last-second score covering 93 yards only because of Campbell's athletic ability. But you wouldn't know it by the headline in the next day's *Daily Missoulian*: "Campbell snares Allen's pass for TD, win with 10 seconds left."

The *Great Falls Tribune* was even more off the mark: "13 seconds left, Allen tosses 93-yard TD pass," the headline blared. Yeah, right. "A desperation 93-yard pass play from quarterback Pokey Allen to halfback Dick Campbell, a couple of seniors climaxing their high school football careers, pulled the Spartans from what looked like a 6-6 tie to the [12-6] victory in the last 10 seconds of the game," said the game account in the *Missoulian*. Technically, it was true, but it was Campbell's catch and run, not my throw, that won the game. That last-second win allowed us to finish 7-2 and in a three-way tie with Kalispell and Butte Central for second place in the Big 10 that year. That kind of stuff happened to me a lot. I wasn't even supposed to play and ended up one of the heroes of the final game. In fact, even though I missed more than half the season I still was named all-state honorable mention and selected as the West's starting quarterback for the 15th East-West Shrine Game, Montana's annual all-star football benefit. (I completed six of 13 passes in a 13-6 loss in the Shrine Game the following summer.) "Pokey Allen came back briefly to show what Missoula might have been had he been able to play after the fourth game of the fall," surmised a local sportswriter at the conclusion of the 1960 season.

Actually, I agree with that assessment. I'm quite certain we would have had a legitimate shot at the state championship had I not missed the second half of the season. Granted, our football team was coming off two mediocre seasons with a combined—and entirely forgettable—6-8-4 record. But we had a new coach in the estimable Thompson, who replaced Royal Morrison, and a strong nucleus of returning players who felt we had the dedication and talent to win the Class AA state title. And I was coming into my own. I had started in the defensive backfield as a sophomore and at both running back and DB my junior year; as a senior I felt well prepared to take over as the Spartans' starting quarterback. Just as we had anticipated, we played well and started the season with victories over

Kalispell, Anaconda, Helena and Billings Senior. But in that fourth game I injured my knee.

Personally, I don't know, but there were those who believed the injury I suffered against Billings Senior might have been inflicted intentionally. To be sure, football is a violent sport and injuries are almost unavoidable, but in the opinion of some members of Missoula's media, the injury that sidelined me was a little more than just "part of the game." "Victory takes big toll [on] Spartans," said the *Missoulian* following our win over Billings. "The Missoula Spartans have paid a high price for their 27-14 Class AA conference victory over the Billings Broncs here late Friday night," said the article. "[Quarterback Pokey] Allen, key to Missoula's offensive and defensive play, fell victim to the roughhouse tactics of the Broncs. On the last play of the first half, a Billings 'tackler' grabbed Allen's face protector and tossed him to the ground, [with] another Bronc piling on. Allen had to be carried off the field with an ankle injury but was able to start the third quarter. Early in the second half Allen was again [tackled] and again a Billings player piled on. This was the last play of the game for Allen and possibly for the rest of the season. His leg is now in a cast with ligaments torn in the knee and ankle." As it turned out, that injury not only ruined the remainder of my senior season in football, it took its toll during the following basketball season, too.

Billings' questionable tactics caused quite a stir in the local media. In fact, two members of the Missoula press, Max Burner, sports editor of the *Daily Missoulian*, and John Campbell, my old Babe Ruth coach and a sportscaster for radio station KYSS, filed official complaints to the president and secretary of the Montana High School Association regarding Billings' "flagrant violation of the rules of sportsmanship." Burner and Campbell cited "unnecessarily rough tactics" by the Broncs involving injuries to me and halfback Rex Hess, both of whom were "severely injured as a result of roughhouse abuse thrown at them."

Is it the press' job to take such action? My answer today would be no; we're talking about an entirely different mind-set among the media of today. Sure, plenty of small-town newspapers and radio stations across America are still "supporters" as much as "reporters" in regard to their local teams. But in larger markets like Boise and Portland, the mentality of the local press is certainly different than when I played high school sports 35 years ago. Is that good or bad? I guess it depends on your perspective.

Chapter 4

State Champs

Winning, whatever the level, is a great source of pleasure and fulfillment. That's probably the main reason basketball was my favorite sport. Sure, there was frustration and disappointment at certain times, but for the most part, my teammates and I from Missoula County High's Class of '61 experienced some of the most exciting and unforgettable moments of our lives playing basketball. From freshmen with a 17-2 record, to Class AA state champions in the 10th grade, to state runners-up as juniors, to state champs again as seniors, we had a marvelous and memorable run.

As early as the start of our ninth-grade season, I had a feeling that the various talents assembled from our class would merge into something special on the basketball court. Part of the reason for that optimism was because of my familiarity with three of my new teammates—John Oblizalo from Roosevelt School and Tom Stage and Larry Schmautz from Willard School. As grade school and junior high athletes, I knew those three as intense baseball and basketball rivals; now we were playing with instead of against each other. My expectations proved to be well-founded as our freshman team, coached by Gene Thompson, averaged 63 points per game en route to that glittering 17-2 record. In Montana, freshman and junior varsity teams from Class AA schools often play the varsity squads of smaller schools, which made our record even more impressive when you consider that some of those wins were against 11th and 12th graders. Oblizalo was our center and leading scorer that first year, averaging 20 points per game while I was second in scoring with a 13 points-per-game average. But I was never much of an offensive threat after my freshman year; my forte was defense, which didn't grab many headlines.

I played center on my eighth-grade team but moved to forward as a freshman because Oblizalo was a natural post player. I remained at forward my sophomore and junior seasons and ended up as a guard my final year because I only grew another two inches, to 6-foot-1, between the eighth and 12th grades. Because I played in the frontcourt most of my career, I never developed the ball-handling skills necessary to be a standout guard. Still, I was a starter on all three teams that went to the state finals under coach Lou "Rock" Rocheleau.

My sophomore year was easily the most enjoyable. Maybe it was because we surprised so many people. With two 10th graders, Oblizalo and me, and junior guard Tim Aldrich in the starting lineup, most observers thought we were too young to contend for the state title. Despite our team's inexperience we won the 1958-59 Big 10 regular-season championship with a 14-4 record and advanced to the state semifinals with a 76-53 playoff win over Helena. Two victories separated our team from the state crown, but the odds still seemed against us. Our main hurdle was two-time defending state champ Butte Public, which defeated our varsity 57-51 the previous year in the title game. Even though we had defeated Butte Public twice during the regular season, the semis and finals were to be held in Butte Civic Center, which gave the Bulldogs a decided home-court advantage. In the semifinals we routed Livingston 75-55 behind Aldrich's 26 points while the Bulldogs trounced cross-town rival Butte Central 78-50 to set up the rematch between the previous year's state finalists.

You know, I played in the Liberty Bowl, I played pro football, I played in some big games in high school, college and the pros, but I still vividly remember that game as the single most tense and exciting event I've ever been associated with as a player. I can still recall that capacity crowd in Butte Civic Center. It was estimated at 8,700, but it seemed like twice that many. It was just an electric atmosphere—what high school sports is all about. Early in the game I scored four of my eight points during an eight-point surge that gave our team a 16-8 advantage. But that was to be our biggest lead of the contest as Butte Public fought back to tie it at 16. After that, neither team gave an inch and there was never more than a four-point difference in the second half. With 2:23 remaining and the game tied at 44, Rocheleau ordered a stall, which worked to perfection. Seniors Jim Pramenko and Dee Pohlman each scored a field goal while we held the Bulldogs to a single free throw for a 48-45 lead in the final minute. Butte Public's Neil McCumber hit a pair of free throws to cut our lead to 48-47, but then the Bulldogs were forced to foul; Oblizalo and Bruce Madsen hit two free throws each to ice the game and we held on for a 52-49 win. It seemed like a tall order to beat Butte Public a third time and win the state championship in a hostile environment, but we did—and the feeling was unbelievable.

I was named all-state honorable mention my junior year, but from a team standpoint, the 1959-60 season was a major disappointment. I mean, most teams would be overjoyed with a state runner-up trophy, but our club felt we could have repeated as state champs were it not for the fact Oblizalo was expelled from school for ... well, let's just say it seemed John couldn't decide which he liked better, beer or basketball. Despite his absence, we finished a respectable 16-8 and reached the title game for the third straight year. The highlight of our season was our 75-73 win over Wayne Estes and Anaconda in the state semifinals. The score was tied seven times in the final quarter before Madsen broke a 71-71 deadlock with a basket and two free throws with less than a minute and a half remaining. With 11 seconds to go, Estes, who finished with 34 points, hit two free throws to cut our lead to 75-73, but Anaconda could get no closer as we held on for the victory. It was an exciting win, but without Oblizalo we were no match for Billings Senior in the championship game the following night and the Broncs bashed us 87-55.

TO BE SURE, reclaiming the state championship and defeating Billings Senior in the semifinals the next year was sweet revenge, but from a personal point of view, my senior year of basketball was fraught with pain and frustration because of my injured knee. I've always been one to put team accomplishments ahead of personal goals, but I couldn't help but feel discouraged throughout that entire season because I never had the kind of year I had hoped for. Sure, winning the state title helped erase much of the disappointment, and I had one of the best offensive games of my career in the finals. But my knee, injured during the preceding football season, never came around and gave me fits all winter; I just wasn't the same player. The injury had already cost me much of my senior season in football, and now it was messing up my last year of basketball; I suffered through a winter of pain and uncertainty, trying to be the player I once was. But it didn't happen. And to make matters worse, I was now playing guard, a position predicated on quickness and mobility, which I didn't have.

I scored 13 points in a preseason tournament game against Livingston and 11 in an early-season loss to Anaconda, but I didn't hit double figures again until the state championship game. I lost confidence in my shot and my defense suffered because of my knee; opponents whom I had dominated defensively the previous three years were now scoring on me. In spite of my limitations, we had enough talent to be in the hunt for the state title and Rocheleau believed my defense was still more than adequate.

So while I concentrated on defense, our other starting guard, a little hotshot junior named Hoyt DeMers, picked up the scoring slack in the backcourt. DeMers, who earned first-team all-state honors at the end of the year, could score from almost anywhere on the floor, and he certainly wasn't shy about trying.

My season of chagrin was shared by Stage, who found himself in a limited role in the second half of the 1960-61 season. Primarily our sixth man, Tom started most of the games at the beginning of the season because Oblizalo was ineligible until the second semester of the academic year. (During his suspension our junior year Oblizalo moved to Deer Lodge to live with his dad; hence he was considered a transfer student and initially ineligible for interscholastic athletics when he returned to Missoula our senior year.) But when Oblizalo rejoined the team in late January of 1961, Stage was relegated to the bench and used sparingly by Rocheleau the rest of the year. Rocheleau was an outstanding coach with a great personality; I really enjoyed playing for him. But Stage, Schmautz (a starting forward) and I were unhappy with his decision to bench Tom. The three of us had played together since our freshman season and always thought that we would be part of a starting unit for the Spartans our senior year. It didn't work out that way, however. (Interestingly, Stage and Schmautz went to Western Montana College together, both taught and coached girls high school basketball in Montana for some 30 years, and both retired from coaching and teaching in 1996.)

Stage had a good shot, but DeMers' was better, and despite my bad knee, my defense and rebounding skills were still better than Tom's. I guess what we found irritating about DeMers being on the floor and Stage being on the bench is that we didn't consider DeMers a "team" player.

Our dissatisfaction notwithstanding, the team began to win when the 6-7 Oblizalo, who went on to play college ball for the University of Utah, returned from his hiatus; gradually all the pieces of the puzzle began to fall into place for another run at the state crown—with Stage, unfortunately, as the odd man out. With Oblizalo and DeMers providing most of the offense, we advanced to the 1961 Class AA final four in Missoula's Montana State University (now the University of Montana) Field House along with Billings Senior, Anaconda and Livingston. Even with Oblizalo back, we knew the state championship would be difficult to attain for two reasons: Billings Senior, our opponent in the semifinals, and Anaconda. The Broncs, after all, were the defending state champs and had whipped our team in the previous year's title game while the Copperheads, led by the Utah State-bound Estes, went unbeaten during the regular season and were considered the pretournament favorites.

Despite the fact we had split our two regular-season games with Billings Senior, we were considered slight favorites over the Broncs for three reasons: First, the tournament was in Missoula. Second, when Billings beat us by 10 points on its home floor early in the season, we were without Oblizalo. Third, in our rematch in Missoula a few weeks later, we crushed the Broncs 84-60 behind Oblizalo's school-record 40 points. (Oblizalo went on to receive a degree in history from Utah; today he drives a truck for a freight line in Las Vegas, where he has lived since 1988.)

But we didn't play like the favorites early in our semifinal game. Billings Senior led throughout most of the second half until we fought back to tie the game at 52 with 40 seconds remaining. Billings worked the clock for a final field goal attempt, but lost the ball out of bounds with 21 seconds remaining. We called a timeout and Rocheleau designed a play to get DeMers open for a final shot. The play failed to materialize, however, and DeMers was caught in a double-team; he passed me the ball near the top of the key with about five seconds left. Billings' Wally Lito, Roger Howell and Ed Bayne, however, were between me and the basket as I drove the lane. As the three defenders converged on me, I flipped an underhand pass to forward Bruce Denison, who hit a short baseline jumper at the buzzer for a 54-52 win. It was Denison's only field goal of the night. Oblizalo had 16 points, Schmautz scored 11 and I had eight. Meanwhile, in the other semifinal, Livingston shocked Estes and Anaconda 70-51, handing the Copperheads their only loss of the year. I guess the Rangers used up all their energy to upset Anaconda, because in the championship game the next night we had a relatively easy time. With Oblizalo scoring 21 points and me adding a career-high 19, we won 79-64 to claim our second title in three years and Missoula County High's sixth state crown overall.

OUR STATE CHAMPIONSHIPS in 1959 and 1961 were the start of a mini-dynasty for Missoula under Rocheleau. Led by DeMers and sophomore forward Mike Lewis, the Spartans reached the state finals in 1962 before losing to Great Falls in the championship game. Then came "The Streak"— 56 consecutive wins over parts of three years (22 wins in 1962-63, 27 in '63-64 and seven more in '64-65). Oddly enough, the Spartans took only one state title during that period because Missoula's school board decided not to let them compete in the 1963 tournament even though they clearly had Montana's best team. The reason: The board said it feared for the safety of Missoula's players and fans. It seems the year before in the state semifinals in Butte, DeMers hit a shot at the buzzer to beat Butte Public 54-53, an outcome that didn't set well with the home team's fans; from what I understand a fracas ensued and the Spartan players had to be escorted to their bus by sheriff's deputies after the game. Because the '63 playoffs were again scheduled in Butte and a recurrence of the ugly scene from the previous year seemed possible, the school board voted to have the unbeaten Spartans forgo the tournament.

The other presumed rationale for the board's ruling, made six months before the 1962-63 season began, was that the Spartans had nothing to prove since they had soundly defeated each league opponent twice during the regular season. Needless to say, it was a controversial decision. In 1964, Lewis' senior year, Missoula again went undefeated and won the state title. Had the school board not made its strange ruling, Missoula most assuredly would have had a streak of seven straight appearances in the state finals (1958 through 1964) and, almost as certain, would have captured four championships during that span.

Rocheleau never forgot his players after their careers ended with the Spartans. Right before I left Missoula to begin college in Salt Lake City, he sent me a letter. It's still in my mom's scrapbook. "I appreciated your hard work, desire and hustle the last four years," he wrote. "You have set a fine example for the young boys who will try to follow in your footsteps. One thing I am convinced that you did in high school was give your team 100 percent all the time. ... The two state basketball championship teams you played on owe much of their success to your defense, hustle and leadership. ... Pokey, I know you are going to be successful in college and I wish you all the luck in the world. Remember, the most important thing is your education, so do a good job with your studies, just as you have always done."

Rocheleau established quite a tradition of basketball excellence at Missoula, and in 1969 he was named the head basketball coach at the University of Montana, his alma mater. I can understand why; he was an outstanding coach and, most important, made basketball fun—a philosophy I have tried to emulate as a coach. Unfortunately, Rocheleau's college coaching fling was brief: In his two years at Montana, 1969-70 and 1970-71, the Grizzlies went 8-18 and 8-16, respectively, and he was replaced by Jud Heathcote. Rocheleau then took a position with Job Corps, a federally funded program for underprivileged youths, in Darby, Montana. He died in February 1980 in Missoula at the age of 54.

SINCE WE WERE kids Jennie and I have been more than just brother and sister; we've been best of friends. We're only 18 months apart in age and have no other siblings, which I guess is part of the reason we've always been so close. But there were times during our high school years when … well, let's just say she didn't always exercise good judgment. I remember once when I was around 17 and she was 16, we got into an argument while I was driving the family car. I don't even recall what we were fighting about, but Jennie decided that she had had enough of my verbal abuse and tried to get out of the car. Problem was we were going about 30 mph at the time, and I had to reach over and grab her to keep her from tumbling out.

That was nothing compared to what she did about a year earlier in another incident involving our car, only this time she was behind the wheel. Adding to the predicament was the fact she didn't have a driver's license. It was a summer afternoon when the two of us were home and our parents were out. Jennie, who was just learning to drive, asked me to give her a ride to the neighborhood grocery store. Now, this store was just a couple of blocks away, so I don't know who was lazier, Jennie or me, because I said, "You kinda know how to drive; take Dad's car … just be careful."

To say Jennie "kinda" knew how to drive is like saying Boise State and the University of Idaho "kinda" have a rivalry going. I mean, her experience behind the wheel was but a few lessons around the block under our dad's strict and watchful instruction. But for some strange reason I suggested she take the car and, even stranger, she did. It was a huge mistake because on her way home she got confused at a stop sign and stepped on the gas pedal instead of the brake and broadsided a parked car, pushing it right up on the lawn in front of Lowell School. And to make matters worse, she panicked, left the scene and ran home. I'll never forget it. So now *I* was in trouble for allowing Jennie to drive the car. As you might imagine, our dad was just a *little* unhappy. I mean, here he was, a local cop with a daughter who drove a car without a license, smashed into another vehicle and fled the scene. He couldn't believe she could be so irresponsible and that I allowed her to do it. He said I was as guilty as she was, and I guess he was right.

As if her harebrained escapades with our car weren't enough, Jennie *really* drove me crazy in high school with her annoying tendency to go out with guys that I didn't, um, particularly care for. "You wanted them [her suitors] to be just like you—boring," she said facetiously (I think) years later. That was easy for her to say; since grade school she was always one of the most popular, outgoing and gregarious members of her class. So, maybe I *was* just a little boring back then. I preferred to think of myself as unassuming and unpretentious; it was sure a heck of a lot better than being cocky and self-important, which was my opinion of some of the guys she dated back then. I've never been certain, but I think she may have done it out of spite. (Maybe she was getting back at me for that time I snitched on her in grade school for talking in class.) At any rate, one of her suitors was Bruce Madsen, and after Madsen went away to college she started dating Hoyt DeMers. I played basketball and baseball with both guys; they certainly weren't adversaries but I didn't consider them among my favorite teammates either. (I should note here that I'm on friendly terms with both of them now.)

AS AN HONOR student and standout athlete I was fairly popular among my peers despite my basic shyness. But throughout my high school years I was hardly what you would call a hell-raiser. In the opinion of some of my schoolmates who liked to drink and carry on, I was probably considered a bit of a "square" (to use a term from that era); with my crew cut and letter sweater, I certainly looked the part. I was the type who stayed out of trouble, but during my freshman year I *did* have a run-in with an older student, a school bully who seemed to have it in for me. His looks, Larry Schmautz remarked years later, resembled those of the TV character Fonzie. Replete with a cigarette pack rolled up in his T-shirt sleeve, black leather jacket and slicked-back hair, his appearance was in stark contrast to mine. Schmautz and I figured that this guy singled me out because he didn't like jocks and I wasn't the confrontational type.

Although I did my best to avoid him, he tried to goad me into a fight more than once. I never sought popularity or recognition among my classmates, but he seemed to resent the fact I was well-liked by most of our fellow students. Anyway, this one time as we were leaving health class he began shoving a classmate of mine named Buddy Zimmerman. Now, Buddy was just a little guy, so I told this bully to "lay off." To which he said, "Do you wanna make something of it?" And I said, "Yeah!" I guess I was just fed up with his guff. We walked outside, took off our shirts and went at it. He got in two pretty good shots, one to the eye and another to the nose. Right then I decided I had had enough; I waded in, grabbed him and threw him to the ground. Just as I was about to beat the crap out of him, he yelled out, "I give up! I give up!" So I let him go and he took off. I won our little set-to, but with a black eye and bloody nose, I looked like the loser. At any rate, that guy never bothered me again and that was the last fight I got into.

I know I have this reputation as a fun-loving guy who likes to live it up and doesn't mind being in the spotlight. But in high school I was just the opposite. It's true I was a member of the National Honor Society and the Key Club and president of the lettermen's club my senior year, but I got involved in those groups because I knew I could still maintain a low profile and wouldn't have to make any speeches. At the time, I really wasn't into personal recognition and did what I could to steer clear of the limelight. That was tough to do, however, because of my success on the athletic field.

I never realized that my desire to stay in the background could be misinterpreted as aloofness—a trait I abhorred—until the summer before my senior year when I attended Boys' State, an annual conference for student leaders sponsored by the American Legion. Designed to teach the participants about government leadership, the statewide conference features a series of mock elections with the "candidates" running for a variety of offices. My roommate at the weeklong conference in Dillon, Montana, was a Missoula High classmate named Dale Schwanke. Schwanke, who is now an attorney in Great Falls, was an honor student, class president our sophomore year, NHS and Key Club president and a real good guy, but not someone I hung around with or knew very well. During the course of the conference we got to know each other better, and after a few days he confessed that he originally wasn't all that pleased when he found out we were going to be roommates. When I asked him why, he said he just would have preferred to room with one of his buddies. Although he never said so, I got the impression he thought I was stuck-up and aloof. That was a real eye-opener because if there was anything I disliked, it was cockiness and arrogance; it still is.

As it turned out, my perception of Schwanke was about as inaccurate as his take on me. At Boys' State I figured he'd be in his element—a key player seeking office and making contacts. But I found out he was almost as uncomfortable in the spotlight as me. "You know," he said. "I don't want to run for any office; I get too nervous in front of groups."

"God, I'm glad you said that," I replied. "I don't want to run for anything either. I'm terrified of public speaking. You have to give all those speeches and I just don't want to do that." I think we found out that we were both just a couple of typical teenagers, shy and unsure of ourselves. I think I learned more from my time with Schwanke that week than anything else I took back from the conference, and we ended up being friends.

Incidentally, four traveling companions, including Jackie Gordon, my girlfriend at the time, and I were involved in a serious car accident on our return trip from that conference. Virgil Walle and Rod Lincoln, two friends from the Superior area, and another guy from Boys' State were in the front seat while Jackie, who had met us in Dillon, and I were in the back. With Walle behind the wheel we were barrelling down the highway between Dillon and Butte when the car ahead of us slowed down to make a right-hand turn. Walle didn't immediately realize that the car had slowed down because we were on a rise in the road that briefly prevented him from see-ing straight ahead. Even so, Walle had a sufficient amount of time to slow down and avoid a collision. The car behind us, however, didn't. That ve-hicle smashed into us; the impact was so great it flipped our car off the road and threw the three occupants in the front seat into the back seat with Jackie and me. The front of the car was crushed and part of the engine was pushed up into the front-seat area. I think the guys in front could have been killed if they hadn't ended up in the back of the car.

Schwanke was in a car behind the vehicle that hit us and showed up at the scene moments later. "When I first saw the wreck I thought for sure that someone had been hurt or killed," he said later. "It's a miracle there weren't any fatalities." Incredibly, no one in our car was seriously injured. From what I recall, an elderly woman in the other vehicle hit her head against the windshield, but even her injury was not critical. A couple of the guys in our car suffered mild concussions and I banged up my knee, but Jackie was unhurt.

Speaking of Jackie, if it weren't for her I probably would have had a very limited social life in high school. She was the one who talked (more like pressured) me into running for freshman class president. From the eighth grade through the middle of our senior year, she pretty much con-trolled my social calendar, such as it was. During the school year we spent a good deal of time together, but during the summer we rarely saw each other because I was playing Legion baseball and her family had a cabin at Flathead Lake. Married to a stockbroker and living in Seattle now, Jackie visited me in the hospital when I was undergoing my cancer treatment in 1995.

Anyway, during the basketball season of our senior year, Jackie de-cided she no longer wanted to go steady. "Sure," I said (perhaps a bit too enthusiastically). We still dated occasionally, and I went out with two other girls from school, Marion Lewis and Darlene Monger, but I was hardly what you would call a ladies' man. I will say, however, that once I stopped dating just one girl, I sort of developed a mental outlook that I'm not so sure is conducive to long-term relationships. I don't mean to imply that I consider dating and physical relationships as some kind of game where a person's emotions and personal feelings aren't important. But after several relationships and two failed marriages, I think I've come to the realization that I'm better at being single than being married. I'm not sure what qualities you need to make a relationship last, but whatever they are, I must not have them. I guess it's just part of my inner nature.

AFTER ALL, PEOPLE change, grow and develop different attitudes and priorities over the years. Take drinking, for example. I didn't drink in high school. Well ... I had a beer at a graduation party, two actually. But that was the first time I ever drank. In school almost everybody drank, mostly beer. And it seemed the girls wanted to be with the guys who were drinking because they were the ones who knew how to party and have fun. Me? I missed a lot of the parties because those who didn't drink often weren't invited. But it wasn't like I stayed holed up in my room either. Missoula was a typical small town, and I can remember "cruisin' the drag" on Higgins Avenue with my friends. There was the usual banter and flirting between the teenage boys and girls who were cruising, but I didn't have the confidence to pursue any of the girls. Still, if I had relaxed just a bit ...

Don't get me wrong. I certainly don't condone underage drinking. Drugs and alcohol are a serious problem in our society; the point I'm trying to make is that if you're held to a set of standards that are unrealistic you're likely to be the object of scorn and almost relentless peer pressure. And you're likely to become resentful. I was told by many teachers, coaches and other adults that if you keep your nose clean, do well in sports and get good grades, you'll be successful. That isn't necessarily true. I don't mean to say you should be some kind of troublemaker or boozehound, but I had plenty of high school classmates and teammates who liked to party and turned out to be highly educated, successful and well-respected members of society. In retrospect, I wish I had had a little more fun in high school, which I eventually did in college.

I finished high school with a 3.6 grade-point average, so I'm pretty sure I could have received some sort of academic scholarship to attend college. My hope, however, was to use my athletic ability to earn a full ride somewhere because my parents didn't exactly have money to burn. But because of my knee injury it wasn't like I was being inundated with scholarship offers. Before I got hurt I received recruitment letters from a number of college football *and* basketball coaches. But after my injury the football offers dwindled to just three—Montana State College (now Montana State University), Utah State and the University of Utah—while the basketball letters disappeared altogether. Despite my success in baseball and basketball, it was apparent that football was my best hope for an athletic scholarship. I mean, even though I was one of the better American Legion baseball players in Montana, I knew I wasn't going to play in the pros after facing Dave McNally. I also thought I was a pretty good high school basketball player, but after my scoring tailed off my senior year I had serious doubts that I could play at the major-college level.

Fortunately, Montana State and the two Utah schools were still interested in my football talents. They hadn't forgotten that I had three really good games at quarterback for the Spartans before I got hurt, and all three were willing to overlook the fact that I missed half of my senior season.

Chapter 5

WAC Wackiness

I don't think I was much different than most 18-year-olds when I went away to college in 1961. Like most teenagers, I could certainly be indecisive and flighty at times. I'm sure Ray Nagel and John Ralston, the head football coaches at Utah and Utah State, respectively, thought as much after a little stunt, albeit unpremeditated, that I pulled on them soon after I joined the Ute football program.

There wasn't much doubt in my mind that I would be playing college football in the state of Utah; I just wasn't sure at which school. I quickly ruled out Montana State for two reasons: I wanted to play in a big-time program and Bozeman was too close to home. That narrowed it down to either Utah or Utah State. I eventually chose the former, but not before a journey into the land of uncertainty by way of Burley, Idaho.

The first person I met from the U of U football program was Ned Alger, the Utes' defensive backfield coach who visited my family and me in Missoula during my senior year in high school; he persuaded me to visit the Salt Lake City school, where I met Nagel. I came away highly impressed by both the school and Nagel, who took me out to breakfast one morning during my visit. Nagel was a real persuasive man, a clean-cut type who said all the right things and reminded me of Bud Wilkinson, the legendary football coach from Oklahoma. As we discussed my future over pancakes and scrambled eggs, I can remember thinking, "Boy, I'm coming here! I'm getting the red-carpet treatment! Just the head coach and me having breakfast together! The way he's talking, I've got a chance to be the starting quarterback my sophomore year!"

By the end of my visit, I had pretty much decided on Utah. But when I visited Utah State a few weeks later I began to have second thoughts because Ralston and the Aggie program were equally impressive.

Still, I chose Utah and signed a letter of intent to play football there.

Back then freshmen were ineligible to play varsity ball, but I reported about a week early and attended the Utes' 1961 season opener against Colorado State. It was then that I began to have serious doubts about my decision. Sophomore quarterback Gary Hertzfeldt threw three touchdown passes against the Rams that day in a 40-0 victory. All of a sudden I started thinking, "Hey, this guy is a sophomore and he's darn good! I might not ever get to play quarterback here!" Almost overnight I had a case of cold feet; suddenly I felt like a lonesome small-town kid in a big city. So I called up this influential Utah State alumnus I knew and explained my predicament. The next thing I knew, there was a cab waiting for me with an airline ticket to Logan. (I know it's only 78 miles from Salt Lake City; I guess this guy was anxious to get me there.)

Now, get this. Like a fool, I took the taxi to the Salt Lake airport and got on the plane, a little propeller job, for the short hop to Logan. But as the plane was preparing to take off I began to realize the error of my ways. So what did I do? Simple … I asked the stewardess if I could get off. Of course she said no, and gave me a look like, Who *is* this idiot? So during the flight I had a chance to ponder my situation, and I started shaking and sweating, wondering what the hell I had gotten myself into and what kind of rules I had broken. To make matters worse, the plane couldn't land in Logan because it was too foggy there, so the flight continued to its next stop—Burley. Now I was *really* sweating because I was basically AWOL from the Utah football program, I had a USU booster wanting me to defect and waiting for me in Logan, and I had somehow ended up in Burley, Idaho, with no clue as to what to do next. And as I got off the plane I quickly realized that my whereabouts were no secret; long-distance phone calls from Nagel, Ralston and my mother awaited my response in the Burley airport office.

I finally did something smart and called my mother first; she talked some sense into me. "Now, Butch," she said reassuringly, "that nice Mr. Alger came all the way to Missoula to see you, and you told that nice Mr. Nagel that you were going to go to school at Utah, so I want you to get on the next bus to Salt Lake and go back there. Mr. Nagel phoned me and told me everything would be OK." So I called Alger (I was too afraid to call Nagel) and told him I was returning to Salt Lake City. But I was still scared. What about the booster in Logan? What about Ralston? I found out soon enough when the bus I had boarded to return to Salt Lake City stopped in Logan. Waiting for me in the depot were Dick Campbell, Wayne Estes and Ralston. Campbell, my high school teammate, was attending Utah State on a football scholarship while Estes, whom I had gotten to know pretty well from our high school sports battles, was a scholarship athlete with the Aggies' basketball program. I was glad to see Campbell and Estes, but I told Ralston I had changed my mind—again—and was returning to Salt Lake City.

Needless to say, my soundness of mind came into question for a while after my return. I remember walking into a room for a team meeting a few days later; as I took my seat I heard a couple of players whisper something like, "Hey, there's that goofy freshman who bolted the team." There was no escape from the embarrassment. An account of my little adventure even made it into the *Salt Lake Tribune* later that week. "'Lost' player ends own tug of war" the headline read. The article didn't have all the facts quite right, but the gist of the story was there: "Pokey Allen, a highly prized prep football player from Montana, will enroll with the rest of the University of Utah frosh gridders Friday morning," the article reported. "But for a time earlier in the week it appeared Pokey would cast his athletic fortunes with Utah State University.

"Allen, who had checked into the University of Utah dormitory, left Monday for Logan by plane, where he talked with the Aggie coaching staff. He returned Tuesday and said, 'I do not want to talk about it.' … In Logan, Ralston said he had talked with Pokey. 'He initiated the conversation with us and we followed it up when he asked about enrolling at USU,' Ralston said. 'His high school teammate, Dick Campbell, is enrolling at USU and we had hoped they would attend school together. Pokey is a fine athlete and student, and any university would be proud to have him in school.'"

In the article, Ralston went on to explain that a student-athlete "must attend a class [which I had not] before he's enrolled at a school. Even his registering doesn't prevent him from changing schools at the last minute." Ralston added, "We tried our best to sell Pokey on Utah State, but when he chose Utah, we were glad he had chosen where he thought his happiness lay. As far as we're concerned, that's it."

Suffice it to say, my college football career got off to an inauspicious start. But once I got my act together I was excited about being part of the Utah football program. My social life, however, was a different story. Like many college freshmen who leave home for the first time, I was ready to "bust loose" and have some real fun. Problem was I was in Salt Lake City—not exactly the party capital of the Intermountain West. Because of the Mormon influence and the fact that the U of U was primarily a commuter school, there wasn't what you would call a thriving nightlife in Salt Lake back then. I was living in a dormitory with several other freshmen football players, and we were all basically in the same boat. Our social life was so pitiful we called ourselves The Pitties. We were all 18 or 19, under the legal drinking age, and only a couple of guys had cars, so we didn't have a lot of off-campus places to go. We would have some beers occasionally, but we were pretty hard up for fun. Our situation was so pathetic that on some Saturday nights our form of dorm-room high jinks bordered on exhibitionism. Some of the more brazen members of the Pitties would play strip poker in front of the window of one of our rooms. Our dorm was on a fairly busy avenue adjacent to the campus, so those who were losing their shirts (or other articles of clothing) risked being exposed to the street below in various stages of undress. Tell me *that* isn't desperate. I mean, we had *nothing* to do. That, I'm afraid, was the only kind of entertainment we could come up with at times.

I think I had maybe three dates my entire first year at Utah, and one of them was a disaster. It all started when a teammate and fellow Missoulian named Ron Plummer talked me into going on a blind date. Plummer, who attended Missoula Loyola and also had been a teammate of mine in Montana's East-West Shrine Game the previous summer, was dating a girl from a Catholic boarding school in Salt Lake. Plummer had made a date to attend some school dance with his girlfriend, but she later called him and said she wasn't going unless he could provide an escort for her friend. Guess who Plummer turned to? I was reluctant, but Ron was insistent, urging me to accompany him because his girlfriend's friend was "a real looker." So I said OK. Well, he lied. I'll be kind and just say it was not a fun evening. But then, not many evenings during my freshman year were.

I didn't get off to a flying start academically either. Like many freshmen, I initially had no idea what I wanted to major in. So when I got to the university, an academic counselor was reviewing my transcripts with me and said, "Shoot. You're a good student and we have an excellent engineering school. You should be an engineer." Sounded good to me. But you know, even though I was an outstanding high school student, I had no note-taking skills, a basic necessity to survive in college. I knew right away that I needed to re-evaluate my academic objectives when I got one of the lowest scores on a paper in a class that was a prerequisite for the engineering program. I eventually switched my major to biology, made the necessary adjustments, and did just fine academically. In fact, I was named to the College Sports Information Directors of America Academic All-America honorable mention football list my senior year.

I originally planned to play both football and baseball at Utah. I was an outfielder and a pitcher for the school's freshman team and returned to the baseball program my sophomore year as a member of the varsity squad's pitching corps. Much like my experience at the plate against Dave McNally in Legion ball a few years earlier, I got a major dose of reality at the collegiate level during the spring of '63 against Arizona State—only this time I was on the mound. During spring break, the Ute baseball team went down to Arizona State for a series against the Sun Devils. I hadn't pitched all that much in the weeks preceding our trip to Tempe. It was still cold in Salt Lake City and we hadn't even practiced outside yet. At the time, ASU had one of the premier college baseball programs in the nation; future major league stars Reggie Jackson, Rick Monday and Sal Bando were among the players who starred for the Sun Devils around that time.

When we squared off with the Sun Devils I think they were ranked second in the nation with a record of 23-3 or something like that. Well, I was the starting pitcher in one of the games, and I struck out the first two batters I faced; all of a sudden I was thinking I was pretty hot shit. Then I walked the next batter. And then the cleanup hitter, I don't remember his name, ripped a line drive through the middle about six feet off the ground. If it had hit me, I think it might have killed me. The ball traveled on a line and hit the center field fence so hard I thought it was going to knock the fence over; I never got another out. I think I pitched in maybe 10 more games, but my arm started bothering me and I was pretty well finished for the year. Besides, the football coaches were pressuring me to concentrate on football because I had a chance to be the starting quarterback in the fall—or so they said.

THE "PLATOON" CONCEPT of having players perform only on offense or defense was already in place in the NFL by the end of the 1950s. But when I played for the Utes from 1961 through 1964 many college players still performed on both sides of the ball. I was recruited as a quarterback and defensive back and was listed as such when I joined the Ute varsity my sophomore year.

As a sophomore I was a starter in the Utes' defensive backfield after the second game of the '62 season, a 35-8 loss to Oregon. In that game Duck running back Mel Renfro, who went on to star as a defensive back for the Dallas Cowboys, ran wild in our secondary, which prompted my promotion to the starting lineup. Two weeks later I had two interceptions in a 35-20 win over Brigham Young; three weeks after that I was named defensive player of the week for my performance, which included a key interception and several tackles, in a 26-8 win over Colorado State. I'd have to say I had a pretty good sophomore year as a DB. I had decent speed and liked to hit people—two necessary ingredients for a good defensive back at that level.

From a team standpoint, however, the '62 season was a disappointment. Utah had a veteran squad, but we never played up to our potential and finished with a 4-5-1 record. In our final game of the year, a 14-11 loss to UCLA, I finally saw some action at quarterback. I gained 30 yards on six carries against the Bruins. Interestingly, my first run from scrimmage went for 12 yards and was captured in a large photograph that appeared in the Salt Lake paper the next day.

The '62 season also marked the Western Athletic Conference's first year of operation. At its inception, the WAC was comprised of Utah, New Mexico, Wyoming, BYU, Arizona State and Arizona. Despite the league's infancy, Utah boasted a strong football program that had been in existence since 1892. During the three years I played for the Utes we had some great players who enjoyed successful careers in the NFL: Tight end Marv Fleming played on Super Bowl winners in Green Bay and Miami; Dave Costa was a standout defensive lineman with Denver, Oakland and Buffalo; Roy Jefferson starred at wide receiver for several years with Pittsburgh, Washington and Baltimore; and Allen Jacobs was a running back for the Packers and New York Giants.

When I reported to camp my junior year I was expected to start in the defensive backfield and serve as second-string quarterback behind Gary Hertzfeldt, who was now a senior. As I originally feared when I witnessed Hertzfeldt's performance against CSU two years earlier, it seemed I was destined to serve as Gary's backup until his playing days at Utah were over. Although I was considered a better runner than Hertzfeldt, he was an outstanding passer, an all-conference selection the previous season and team captain that year. Still, I was pretty optimistic that I would get to see some action at quarterback during the 1963 season. As it turned out, I saw plenty. When our season began Hertzfeldt was recovering from eye surgery, and although Gary was ready to play I got the nod to start at quarterback in our opener against Oregon State. Unfortunately, neither I nor the team performed well against Tommy Prothro's Beavers and we lost 29-14.

I started at quarterback in our next game, a 10-9 loss to Idaho in Boise. (Because of UI's large alumni base in Ada County, the Vandals regularly played "home" games in Boise back then.) It was hotter than blazes that day, around 100 degrees. The game was played on the BSU campus near where the Student Union now stands. The reason I remember that game is because I don't remember much. Early in the first quarter I got nailed by Vandal linebacker Dick Litzinger; it was one of the hardest hits I ever took. It dented my helmet and just knocked me silly. I vaguely remember wobbling back to the bench and Hertzfeldt pleading, "Pokey, you gotta shake it off! I can't play quarterback *and* safety!" But I was done for the day. In fact, I remember very little until after we were back in Salt Lake City. In the game's closing moments Hertzfeldt drove our offense to a touchdown that cut Idaho's lead to 10-9, but running back Ron Coleman was stopped short of the goal line on the two-point conversion attempt with 36 seconds left and the Vandals prevailed.

Despite my head injury and the fact we were 0-2 with me as the starting quarterback, I drew the starting assignment again in our next game at New Mexico. It was a daunting task. The game was in Albuquerque and the Lobos were the defending WAC champs and 12-point favorites. But in one of the biggest upsets of the season, we stunned UNM 19-6. I shared the quarterbacking duties with Hertzfeldt and rushed for 48 yards on eight carries, including a 23-yard touchdown run on an option play for the game's first score. I also threw a two-yard TD pass to Jefferson in the fourth quarter.

In our next game against Brigham Young, Hertzfeldt and I again split the QB duties. We were favored to beat the Cougars at home, but BYU's defense was outstanding and we held a 7-6 lead in the fourth quarter. With our slim lead looking vulnerable, Mike Davis intercepted a pass by BYU's Phil Brady on our five-yard line. We proceeded to march 95 yards and I finished the drive with a one-yard TD run that secured the win. The hold on the extra-point attempt was bobbled, but I picked up the loose ball and threw a two-point conversion to Jefferson to round out the scoring in the 15-6 victory.

We routed Colorado State 48-14 at home the following week for our third straight win, but then I reinjured my bad knee the next week during a 26-23 loss to Wyoming. I didn't play in our next two games, a 30-22 loss to Arizona State and an 8-7 setback to Army. I returned for our final two games, a 35-22 loss to Cal and a 25-23 upset win over Utah State in Logan. That final game creates an interesting trivia question: What two future Boise State head football coaches were on the field that day? The answer: USU's first-year head coach Tony Knap and me. (Knap served as an assistant with the Aggie program before he was promoted to head coach following the 1962 season when John Ralston took the head coaching job at Stanford. Knap went on to become a coaching icon, deservedly so, during his eight years in Boise. BSU posted an amazing 71-19-1 record under Knap from

1968 through 1975, winning the Big Sky championship and advancing to the NCAA Division II playoffs in each of his final three years with the Broncos. He took the head coaching job at UNLV after the '75 season. After nine years at Stanford, in which he led the Cardinal to two Rose Bowl wins, Ralston coached the NFL's Denver Broncos and USFL's Oakland Invaders. A member of the College Football Hall of Fame, Ralston concluded his 40-year coaching career at the end of the 1996 season when he stepped down as the head coach at San Jose State.)

I also remember that game against the Aggies because it was the day after President Kennedy was assassinated. At first we weren't even sure whether we were going to play the game at all. On the afternoon of November 22, 1963, we boarded our team bus, drove to Ogden and spent the night there while officials from the two schools discussed whether or not we should play the game the next day. Finally, it was decided we would play and the bus continued on to Logan. Led by quarterback Bill Munson, who starred for Los Angeles and Detroit during a 16-year career in the NFL, USU had an outstanding team that year. Going into the season finale, the Aggies were 8-1 and had clobbered their victims by an average score of 35-6. We were an unimpressive 3-6 and decided underdogs. In the fourth quarter, however, Hertzfeldt hit Davis with a 35-yard touchdown pass and our defense made a goal-line stand at the end of the game to preserve the upset win. It was a strange game; Kennedy's death cast a pall over the stadium. There was no band playing, no excitement in the air. We were pleased with the win, but it was a solemn finish to a disappointing season.

MY SENIOR YEAR began on a positive note when Jefferson and I were elected team co-captains by our teammates during the spring drills that preceded the 1964 season. I considered it an honor to earn that distinction along with Jefferson, who would go on to earn consensus All-America honors as a split end that fall; not only was Roy a great football player, he is an outstanding person. There was another reason why I was excited about my senior year: I figured I was the automatic choice as the Utes' No. 1 quarterback. My rivalry with Hertzfeldt was always friendly and we ended up being good friends, but I must say I was pleased when Gary finally graduated. I figured I would step right in and assume control of the offense with Rich Groth, a fellow senior who played mostly defense the previous year, serving as my backup.

We got off to a great start with a 16-0 win over two-time defending WAC champ New Mexico in the season opener. As expected, I started at quarterback against the Lobos and had a good game with a 14-yard touch-down run and a 49-yard scamper in the first half. But our defense was the real story—as it would be the entire season. UNM could muster only 119 yards total offense to our 401 yards. The following week, however, we got hammered by Missouri 23-6 in Columbia and I had an atrocious game at quarterback, going something like two for 12 with two interceptions.

That led to the low point of my senior year. Let me preface this by saying that as a recruiter and tactical coach Nagel was first-rate, but I didn't care much for the way he kept his distance from his players once they joined the program; he rarely spoke to any of us on a one-to-one basis. Because I was primarily a defensive back when I joined Utah's football program, most of my dealings were with Ned Alger and Chuck Chatfield, another defensive coach. Fortunately, Alger was accessible and helpful, the kind of coach you could confide in. In Nagel's defense, I would add that his style was how most coaches dealt with their players in the early '60s. (As a head coach, I don't believe in being detached and impassive when dealing with my players; that just isn't my style. Of course you can't be buddy-buddy with them, but you still need to be approachable.)

Anyway, Nagel and some of his assistants had this disconcerting habit of ignoring players who had fallen out of favor, and I started getting the cold shoulder right after the loss to Missouri. Eventually, Nagel told me he was benching me as quarterback in favor of Groth. Needless to say, I was pretty upset, not only because of the demotion but because of the way I was being treated. I mean, here I was, team captain and a senior and my head coach rarely speaks to me except to inform me that I'm no longer the starting quarterback. I even cried because I had worked so hard to earn the starting quarterback position. At least I knew they weren't going to bench me on defense because I was still one of the team's best DBs. In fact, I honestly think our three-man alignment of Frank Andruski, C.D. Lowery and me was one of the best defensive secondaries in the West, if not the nation, that year. I know that sounds like bragging, but we fin-ished the season with the statistics to back it up. Andruski, Lowery and I weren't fast, but we were tenacious. "Don't worry about our slowness, coach," I remember saying to Alger with a laugh during the season. "Once our opponents get inside our 20, they have less room to maneuver, and their speed doesn't do them any good. That's when we stop 'em."

Our next game was against Idaho in Salt Lake, and I figured I would be spending most of my time on defense. But our offense was sluggish and Groth was ineffective in the first two quarters, completing just one pass in seven attempts as we battled the Vandals to a scoreless tie through the first half. I started the second half at quarterback and promptly led our offense on an 80-yard drive, capping the march myself with a one-yard TD run. Our defense continued to blank the Vandals, and in the fourth quarter I threw touchdown passes of 28 yards to Merlin Driggs and two yards to Jerry Pullman for a 22-0 win.

I was back in Nagel's good graces and started at QB the next week against Wyoming in Laramie. Our defense was excellent again as we limited the Cowboys to 10 first downs and 237 yards total offense, but we lost a 14-13 heartbreaker when Jefferson, who also served as our place-kicker, missed an extra point that would have tied the game in the third quarter. I completed eight of 13 passes for 149 yards including a 46-yard TD throw to Jefferson, but it wasn't enough.

With the exception of the Missouri game, I thought my performance at quarterback had been satisfactory, but after four games we were 2-2 and our offense was still sluggish. Our offense didn't fare much better the following week, but we did manage to down Colorado State 13-3 in Fort Collins. Our defense, on the other hand, was exceptional again. We limited the Rams to 184 yards total offense and our secondary collected four interceptions.

With our offense still struggling Nagel decided to hand the quarterback position back to Groth. The following week we beat Arizona State 16-3 in Salt Lake, ending the Sun Devils' 12-game winning streak and holding them to their lowest point total in 76 contests. I started at defensive halfback and didn't play quarterback until four minutes were left in the game. It was after that contest that we began to realize just how good our defense was. With future NFL running backs Tony Lorick and Charley Taylor on ASU's talent-laden offense, holding the Sun Devils to a single field goal was quite an accomplishment.

We were on a roll now. We whipped Texas Western 41-0 in El Paso the following week to improve our record to 5-2; in those five victories our defense had yet to yield a touchdown. That game was followed by a 47-13 rout of BYU; our defense did an effective job against Virgil Carter, the Cougars' star quarterback, and Allen Jacobs rushed for 115 yards and four touchdowns. Groth started at quarterback while I finished up with a 20-yard TD pass to Driggs late in the game.

With the offense playing well under Groth's direction and our defense running on all cylinders with me in the secondary, it became evident that I was more valuable to the team at defensive back than at quarterback. *Salt Lake Tribune* sports editor John Mooney said as much in a column he wrote at midseason:

"Pokey Allen has made a sacrifice for the good of the Redskins," Mooney wrote. "Allen gave up his role as quarterback for a defensive post as a team contribution. ... As a Utah soph, Pokey played mostly defense as he earned his spurs. Last season, he started at quarterback, but an injury shelved him and Gary Hertzfeldt came on to earn all-conference quarterback honors. As a senior Pokey figured to come into his own. But after a few games it was obvious Allen was more valuable as a defensive man than an offensive passer. As team captain, Allen was willing to play where he could do the most good, even if it meant sacrificing a lot of personal glory."

Several years later, Alger, who went on to become Utah's associate athletic director, made a similar comment to a reporter that meant a lot to me. "We were a better football team with Pokey on defense," he remarked. "He was a very smart player. Having him in the defensive secondary was like having another coach on the field."

Our next test was California and its star quarterback Craig Morton. Although we were on a four-game winning streak and the Golden Bears were 3-5, Cal was still the clear favorite in our showdown in Berkeley. Morton, after all, was one of the nation's premier quarterbacks and we had never beaten the Bears in three previous tries. But our defense was up to the task again and we battled to a scoreless tie going into the final quarter. We finally broke the deadlock and took a 6-0 lead early in the fourth period when Ron Coleman scored on a six-yard TD run. With five minutes remaining, Morton, who had thrown at least one touchdown pass in 16 straight games, tried to engineer a winning drive from the Cal 20-yard line. Having thrown 96 consecutive passes without an interception, Morton finally threw one—to me. Defensive lineman Dario DeBenedetti forced Morton to hurry his throw and I picked off the pass at the Bears' 44-yard line and ran it back to the 18. Four plays later Coleman scored from four yards out and Groth hit John Pease for the two-point conversion to clinch the victory.

Our 14-0 upset was called "one of Utah's greatest victories in recent years" by the *Salt Lake Tribune* and "Utah's proudest hour in Bay Area competition" by the *San Francisco Examiner*. Morton, who went on to star in the NFL and lead both Denver and Dallas to the Super Bowl, completed 22 of 37 passes and drove his team inside our 20-yard line six times, only to be denied by our defense.

With a 7-2 record going into our regular-season finale against Utah State, talk of a bowl bid had already begun. "Bowl-conscious Utes hammer Bears, 14-0," blared one headline after the win in Berkeley; both the

Salt Lake Tribune and United Press International speculated that an offer to play in the Sun Bowl would be coming our way—especially if we could beat the Aggies. All that did, however, was give Tony Knap and his players more incentive; I'm sure they would have liked nothing more than to ruin our chances of appearing in a bowl with a season-ending victory in Ute Stadium.

Funny thing, not all of our players were very excited about the prospect of playing in a bowl; the thought of an additional month of football practices, which would be necessary if we were to receive a bowl invitation, was unappealing. The reason was assistant coach Bob Watson. He was just a mean person, plain and simple. Lucky for me and the other backs, he coached the linemen, so I didn't have to deal with him very much. But many of the lineman just didn't like him, and we all knew that if we beat Utah State and went 8-2 we would probably go to a bowl game. In fact, during the week of practice preceding the USU game, some of the players were chanting, "Seven and three and the Christmas tree!" meaning they didn't want to beat the Aggies and extend our season any longer. When the coaches became aware our discord, they met with the players the Wednesday before the USU game. They admitted that it had been a long, tough season; they went on to say that we had done a great job all year and that if we managed to win Saturday's game and play in a bowl game, they would promise to conduct practices that were more relaxed. Well, we won—and they lied.

As expected, the game against Utah State was a hard-fought affair. The Aggies' record was only 5-3-1, but they had several outstanding athletes, including future NFL players Roy Shivers, Ron Sbranti and Earsell Mackbee. I think it was only appropriate that we won that game on the strength of our defense. We intercepted four passes by USU quarterback Ron Edwards, including two by me, and recovered three fumbles en route to the 14-6 win. We jumped out to a 7-0 lead in the opening quarter on a 51-yard touchdown pass from Groth to Pease, and Jacobs added a 14-yard TD run in the third period for a 14-0 lead before the Aggies averted a shutout on an 11-yard scoring pass from Edwards to Shivers.

The win gave us an 8-2 record, Utah's most successful season in 11 years and Ray Nagel's best mark in six years as coach. We captured a share of the 1964 WAC championship with New Mexico and Nagel was later named United Press International Coach of the Year. Our defense had four shutouts, yielded only 62 points—an average of just over six points per game—and finished the regular season ranked sixth in the nation. We awaited a bid from the Sun Bowl in El Paso.

BUT INSTEAD THE invitation came from the Liberty Bowl—not exactly the granddaddy of 'em all, but a bowl game nonetheless. Utah hadn't been to a bowl in 26 years, so I don't imagine the coaches were too picky. We were pitted against West Virginia, a member of the Southern Conference with a 7-3 record, in a game that would be televised nationally December 19, 1964, from Atlantic City, New Jersey. The first interesting bit of news about this game was that it would be held indoors. The inaugural Liberty Bowl drew 36,000 fans to Philadelphia Stadium in 1959, but the game was becoming a financial failure as wintry weather kept attendance figures down during the next four years. (Bad weather on the East Coast in December? Gee, what a surprise.) Thus the bowl's promoters decided to move the game inside the famed Convention Hall in Atlantic City for what *The Sporting News* called "the first indoor major college postseason football game in history."

Now, in this day and age of carpeted playing surfaces and domed stadiums, indoor football games are a common part of contemporary American sports. But our contest with West Virginia was held four months before the first indoor major league baseball game was played in Houston's Astrodome. And four *years* before the Houston Oilers became the first pro football team to play in an indoor stadium. Furthermore, the nation's first permanent indoor facility for a college football program, Idaho State's Holt Arena, wouldn't become a reality for another six years. (I'm not a football historian, but the only other indoor college or pro game of any significance that I'm aware of before our game in '64 was the first playoff game in NFL history. It took place in Chicago Stadium between the Bears and the Portsmouth Spartans in December 1932 because of bitter cold and heavy snow. I read that the field was only 80 yards long and the arena walls butted against the sidelines.)

As we prepared for our Liberty Bowl battle with West Virginia, the media noted several common traits between the two teams. We were both 4-6 the previous year and both teams started the 1964 season with 2-2 records. West Virginia, which had defeated a good Kentucky team and Sugar Bowl-bound Syracuse during the regular season, was considered a clear-cut favorite by the East Coast media. But we were confident. A few days before our showdown with the Mountaineers, the *Tribune* ran a photo of the team boarding our charter plane for the flight to Atlantic City. I read with great interest the final lines of the article that accompanied the photo:

"In a minor switch in strategy, Nagel indicated that captain Ernest 'Pokey' Allen might get more of a shot on offense in this his final collegiate game," the article stated. "Allen took over as a defensive back and helped Utah to its fine defensive record. Richard Groth, who sparked the team at quarterback in the last half of the season, will alternate with Allen." I wasn't sure why Nagel had made that comment to the *Trib*, but I sure wasn't complaining. Looking back, I think when all was said and done, the coaching staff had confidence that I would make the right decisions at quarterback.

The players on our team were pretty relaxed and having a good time on the East Coast as we prepared for the game. In fact, it was the most relaxed we had been all season. I think one reason was because as a visiting team from the West in a bowl game, we were in the public eye a lot more than we were used to and Watson couldn't bully us anymore. He couldn't punish us, run us or hit us—like he was inclined to do under normal circumstances—without serious media scrutiny.

I hate to say this, but the sixth annual Liberty Bowl was kind of cheesy. There was a small crowd, 6,059, and it was just plain weird playing football inside. At the time, Atlantic City's Convention Hall was billed as the largest facility of its kind in the world—the venue for the annual Miss America pageant and the building where President Lyndon Johnson had accepted his party's nomination at the Democratic national convention four months earlier. But as the site for a college football game, it left a lot to be desired. The playing surface consisted of three inches of sod over one inch of burlap on the building's concrete floor, and the end zones were eight feet smaller than normal. One end line was smack up against the platform where LBJ and other Democratic leaders stood the previous August. White vapor lights, originally installed for TV coverage of the Democratic convention, provided the lighting, giving the game an almost surreal atmosphere.

The game itself, however, was business as usual for the Utes; we were there to win a football game. As predicted, I started at quarterback, and things immediately fell into place. Jefferson kicked field goals of 32 and 35 yards to get us off to a 6-0 lead in the second quarter. Then I scored on an 11-yard run and Coleman added a brilliant 53-yard dash to give us a 19-0 lead at halftime.

We were in complete control when I went back on defense in the second half. In the third quarter I was covering a West Virginia receiver when Mountaineer quarterback Allen McCune got hit as he released a pass; I couldn't have dropped the ball if I had wanted to as it fluttered into my waiting arms. A few minutes later Andy Ireland, a senior running back, added a 47-yard touchdown run for a 25-0 lead. West Virginia scored late in the third period to avert a shutout. We got one more score when Groth hit Bill Morley with a 33-yard touchdown pass.

Our 32-6 win in the Liberty Bowl gave us seven consecutive wins and a 9-2 record. Coleman, who is now a vice president at the U of U, had a great game. His long touchdown run was part of a 154-yard performance that should have given him the MVP trophy. But my overall effort—five of 11 passes for 72 yards, five rushes for 28 yards and an interception—impressed the voters and I was named MVP. We picked off four more interceptions against the Mountaineers, giving us 27 for the year. Lowery had one of our thefts, giving him eight, which tied him for the most in the nation that year. I finished with five. And as the finishing touch on what had to be one of the tackiest bowl games ever played, Ed McMahon, a West Virginia graduate, presented our team with the winner's trophy.

It was a very satisfying triumph and a great way to end my college career. Our relatively unknown team traveled east and showed a national television audience that we knew how to play football in the West. "The Utes amazed the [East Coast] writers who had been impressed by West Virginia's victory over Syracuse's Sugar Bowl team and Kentucky of the Southeast Conference," wrote the *Salt Lake Tribune's* Mooney in his column the next day. "Utah and Western Athletic Conference football hit a new high point because a Utah victory before the nation's fans improved the football image of every team in the area."

Mooney also briefly mentioned me in that same column. In describing the scene in the press box during the game, Mooney said that one of his fellow reporters asked him, "What pro team drafted Pokey Allen?" The writers, Mooney wrote, "couldn't believe no pro club wanted Pokey."

Chapter 6

Canadian Clubs

C ould I have played in the NFL? Probably not. I'd like to think I was a pretty decent college football player, but when you start talking NFL, you're obviously talking about the best of the best. Although I wasn't selected in the NFL draft after the 1964 season, the Dallas Cowboys did approach me about signing a contract as a free agent. I was flattered, but realistically I knew the NFL summer camps, including Dallas', would be filled with players just like me: long on determination but short on natural ability.

If Dallas coach Tom Landry had been making his roster decisions based solely on a player's instinct and desire, maybe I would have had a shot. But in the NFL it's all about talent, speed, size and strength. I don't think I was deficient in any of those departments, but I wasn't at the level needed to play in the NFL. When I finished my career at Utah I was 6-foot-1, 185 pounds, big enough to play quarterback or defensive back in the NFL. But I didn't quite have the arm to play the former and I wasn't quite fast enough for the latter.

I might not have been good enough for the NFL, but I still thought I could play professional football; so did the British Columbia Lions. After the 1964-65 school year I signed a contract for $10,500 a year, plus a $2,000 signing bonus, with the defending champs of the Canadian Football League. (I didn't have quite enough credits to graduate from the University of Utah in 1965 and planned to complete the requirements for my degree in the off-season.) Taking a shot at the NFL was tempting, I told the *Missoulian*, but I thought my chances were better in the CFL. "I decided I would rather go to Canada where they give an all-around athlete more of a chance to play," I told my hometown newspaper a few days before I left for the Lions' training camp. "I don't have blazing speed and I figure things will work out better at Vancouver. It's a great city and has a great team. I feel it's the best club to go with in the Canadian league." The story in the

Missoulian was accompanied by a photograph of my mom and me as we looked over a road atlas to map out my trip to Vancouver. While the article focused on my immediate future, it also foreshadowed the career path I would eventually travel—a journey that would extend into four decades. When asked about my long-term plans, I told the reporter, "I would like to coach at the college level."

British Columbia had captured the Grey Cup, the CFL's equivalent of the Super Bowl, in 1964; unfortunately the Lions were beginning a downward slide when I joined them in the summer of '65. (Some of my so-called friends still take great delight in pointing out that the Lions' decline and my arrival started at just about the same time.) Actually, the reason for B.C.'s fall was a combination of aging and injured players and an ongoing battle between star quarterback Joe Kapp and team management. Kapp was a natural-born leader, but I also thought he was a disruptive force on the Lions.

Unlike the NFL, which had gone to the platoon system more than a decade earlier, the CFL still used many players on both offense and defense. I earned a starting spot in the defensive backfield and also served as the backup quarterback to Kapp, who would go on to lead the Minnesota Vikings to the Super Bowl four years later. Interestingly, I would also be an assistant coach under Kapp at the University of California 17 years later.

Given the success of the previous year, the Lions' 1965 season was nothing short of a disaster. With alarming speed they fell on hard times and finished fourth in the CFL's five-team Western Conference with a 6-9-1 record. I hate losing as much as the next guy, but from a personal perspective I had a bang-up rookie year. In fact, my "hard-hitting" style caught the attention of Vancouver sportswriter Jim Brooke before the season even started. "The rookie defensive back's slashing hitting in scrimmages has provided the training camp with one of its minor sensations," Brooke wrote. "Allen earned his starting defensive post by delivering some jolting shots at the likes of [flanker] Sonny Homer and fullback Bob Swift. Allen came like a thunderbolt to 'stick' Swift right on the goal line and prevent a scrimmage TD earlier in the week."

I ended up with four interceptions and was one of the team's leading tacklers in 1965. In fact, I was so pleased with my first-year performance that I briefly reconsidered taking a stab at the NFL. But by then I had fallen in love with the city of Vancouver. And besides, the NFL's salaries weren't a whole lot more than the CFL's back then.

To provide an alternative to what the NFL generally offers, the CFL traditionally features more of a wide-open brand of football. To that end, the CFL has several variations to the rules that govern football in the United States—12 players, three downs to make 10 yards, a longer (by 10 yards) and wider (by 11 and a half yards) field, deeper end zones, legal motion by backs and receivers before the snap, and one point for missed field goals that aren't returned out of the end zone. Those differences were no big deal, but there was one alteration that I did have a problem with: punt returns without blockers. The reason for my objection? I was the Lions' punt returner my rookie year. Think about it … one poor schmuck with 12 opposing players flying down the field *unimpeded* trying to break him in half! I mean, what kind of insanity is that? True, the punt returners were allowed a five-yard buffer zone until they caught the ball, but so what? It was still one against 12! Despite the foolishness of it all, I led the Lions with 55 punt returns for 262 yards and a 4.7 yards-per-return average that year. A year or so after I left the Lions, the team's top punt-return man was Jerry Bradley. Bradley, a Vancouver stock promoter who has been one of my best friends for the past 30 years, had the right idea when he fielded punts: He would catch the ball and head for the sidelines. The rule was changed to allow blocking (what a novel idea!) in 1975.

After my first season with B.C. I returned to the University of Utah for one quarter to finish up my degree, a bachelor of science in biology. In 1966 I saw action at quarterback in two exhibition games for the Lions because Kapp was injured. (Pete Ohler eventually became the Lions' other QB and I returned to the defensive backfield.)

There was one occasion early in the season, however, when I thought I was going to start at quarterback. Kapp and I roomed together on road trips, and on a trip to Toronto to play the Argonauts, Kapp snuck out of our hotel after curfew the night before a game. Blacky Johnston, one of the assistant coaches, came into our room to do a bed check. Kapp had a reputation as one who liked to gallivant, so Johnston was suspicious from the start. "Where's Joe?" he asked. "Um, he's in the bathroom," I said. Johnston: "Can I see him?" Me: "Uh, I think he's in the shower." Johnston: "I don't hear the shower running." Me (starting to panic): "Um, maybe he's indisposed." Johnston (peering into the empty bathroom): "Indisposed my ass! Goddamit, Pokey! You're covering for him, aren't you! You better come clean or you'll be in trouble, too!" Me: "Honest, Blacky! I must have been asleep! I don't know where he is!"

Johnston left and Kapp eventually returned about 5 a.m. Later that morning head coach Dave Skrien and Johnston called me into Skrien's room. "Kapp's benched," Skrien said. "You're starting at quarterback tonight." I said, "OK," but I wanted to blurt out, "Oh shit, you gotta be kidding!" Just before the opening kickoff, however, Kapp was reinserted as the starting QB. "Well, this is interesting," I said to myself. It got even more interesting when Johnston was fired a week later.

Like I said, Kapp was a leader among his fellow players, but his stormy relationship with management and Skrien undermined the coaching staff's authority and hurt our chances of winning. Nothing went right that year as Kapp's petulance as well as injuries to star players such as linebacker Tom Brown and running back Willie Fleming continued to plague the team. Skrien was fired after the fourth game and replaced by interim coach Ron Morris for one game before Jim Champion took over on a permanent basis. We finished in last place with a dismal 5-11 mark.

British Columbia fared no better the next year under Champion. The Lions were in the throes of a precipitous plunge that saw them again finish in the cellar with a woeful 3-12-1 record. And as often happens when a team struggles, B.C. made a number of personnel changes that year. In the Canadian Football League each team is required to have 17 import and 17 non-import players on its roster. The details of the rule are a bit complicated, but the bottom line is that the non-import players (Canadian residents and others who meet certain requirements) are often at a premium. Thus when a team seeks to move players around, as was the case with the Lions in '67, import players like me are usually more expendable. With the team going nowhere fast, Champion decided to make some changes and I was released after the fourth game.

I got picked up on waivers by Edmonton and played DB for the Eskimos for two games but got cut again. I knew Edmonton and I weren't meant to be after that second game; ironically, that contest was against B.C. It was just before halftime and the game was still close when I got burned on a long pass by wide receiver Jim Young for a touchdown. I was right with Young as quarterback Bernie Faloney lofted the pass, but then Young blew by me, caught the ball and scored easily. I kind of followed him into the end zone with a jog as the play ended. I should have just kept jogging—over the fence, out of the stadium, down the street to the closest bar in downtown Edmonton for a beer because I knew I was history. I desperately needed my paycheck, however, so I returned to the bench and actually stayed in the game for the second half. But, as expected, the Eskimos sent me packing the next day.

I THOUGHT MY playing days were over, but I found new life in another CFL—the Continental Football League. I had returned to Vancouver after being cut by Edmonton because I still had an apartment there and the Lions owed me one more paycheck. While I was in the Lions office to pick up my money, one of the assistant coaches saw me wandering the halls and asked if I was interested in playing anymore football. He said the Norfolk Neptunes of the Continental Football League had recently lost two defensive backs to injuries and were looking for a replacement or two to help them in their drive for the league championship. I wasn't even sure where Norfolk, Virginia, was, but after a couple of telephone conversations with Neptunes head coach Gary Glick I found out, and I was on my way—a trip of more than 3,000 miles. (Here's an interesting bit of trivia regarding Glick: A defensive back from Colorado A&M, now Colorado State, he was selected by Pittsburgh as the NFL's No. 1 draft choice in 1956.)

Founded in the mid-60s, the Continental Football League was a forerunner of the World Football League of the 1970s and the United States Football League of the 1980s—both ill-fated attempts to compete with the mighty NFL. But the Continental Football League had even more going against it. Unlike the WFL, which formed after the AFL-NFL merger in 1970, the CFL originally had two other pro football leagues to compete against (three if you count the other CFL). And unlike the USFL, the Continental Football League did not have a TV contract or incredibly wealthy investors like Donald Trump to help it along. Although it billed itself as America's third pro football league, the CFL was not much more than a hodgepodge of floundering franchises playing many of its games on poorly lighted fields in front of sparse crowds. Two exceptions were the Neptunes and the Orlando Panthers, both of whom enjoyed considerable support from their communities. It was no coincidence that they were also the CFL's two best teams.

The Continental Football League was an interesting collection of players and places. Our opponents included the Charleston Rockets, Pottstown Firebirds, Wheeling Ironmen, Hartford Charter Oaks (whatever *those* are) and Richmond Rebels—not exactly the most "happening" places in the Eastern U.S. Granted, the league also had some big-city franchises that played in modern stadiums—the Toronto Rifles, Montreal Beavers, Philadelphia Bulldogs and Brooklyn Dodgers among them—but those clubs were on equally shaky financial ground. When I arrived to play for the Neptunes with about eight games remaining in the 1967 season, the league was already starting to crumble. I remember playing a game in Montreal and then learning that the Beavers had folded a few days later.

As expected, Norfolk had a successful regular season, and we earned the right to host Orlando in the championship game. The Neptunes used

Old Dominion University's Foreman Field, a stadium that seated 27,000, and since we had averaged around 17,000 or 18,000 per game and once drew 20,400 the previous year, the team's owners expected a large crowd for the title game with the Panthers. Similarly, the players anticipated a hike in their cut from the gate receipts. But when management balked at giving the players an increase from their usual take, we went on strike the week of the game. Our ringleader was quarterback Dan Henning, who went on to coach the Atlanta Falcons from 1983-86. Well, the strike backfired on both the players and management. We eventually gave in and ended the strike about 48 hours before the game; therefore we had just one day to prepare for the Panthers, who ended up beating us in a close game, 20-14 I believe the score was. In addition, the crowd was a big disappointment. It seemed many of the local fans were disillusioned with the strike, and with only two days' notice that the game was indeed going to be played, many of them apparently opted to make other plans for that day.

I didn't make a whole lot of money playing for the Neptunes, but I sure had a lot of fun—especially with a fellow defensive back from Wake Forest named Pete Manning. As many single men in their 20s are wont to do, Manning and I would frequent some of the watering holes in Norfolk and on the road. Now, if you're trying to impress some girl in a bar, you would think that telling her you were a pro football player would help your chances. But for Manning, that wasn't good enough. He and I fabricated this story in which he was a graduate student in sociology from Harvard and I was a millionaire's son from Alaska. He was playing for the Neptunes to conduct research on his master's thesis—some kind of examination, he would claim, "of professional football's impact on the sociological tendencies on blah-blah-blah ..."

He didn't really enjoy playing football, he would say (amazingly with a straight face); he was doing it for the intellectual stimulation and betterment of mankind. Me? My trumped-up story didn't require quite as much imagination or guile. I was a rich kid playing football on a lark whose dad was some kind of gold-mining tycoon from Alaska. But you know what? Sometimes it worked. I'll tell you one thing: During my stay with the Neptunes my love life improved dramatically when I was with Manning.

While playing in the two CFLs in 1967, I eventually came to the realization that my pro football career was destined to be neither long nor lucrative. So during that time I started to work on getting a stockbroker's license through a correspondence course out of Vancouver. After the Neptunes' loss to Orlando I moved back to Vancouver, received my license in January 1968, and worked as a stockbroker through the first five or six months of that year. That spring I was offered the job as defensive back coach at Simon Fraser University, a small four-year school in Burnaby, a suburb of Vancouver. The school was only five years old and the Clansmen football program had been in existence for only three years, but I thought the position would be a good starting point into the coaching profession. Besides, I really needed a job because I decided I wasn't all that interested in being a broker. My first contract at SFU was for $8,200. We went 4-4 that fall.

I thoroughly enjoyed coaching, but in the back of my mind I still wasn't ready to call it quits as a player. After one year as an assistant with Simon Fraser, I tried a comeback with the Lions in the summer of 1969. SFU head coach Lorne Davies was good enough to leave my job open for me in case I got cut, which turned out to be a good thing. The Lions posted a record of 4-11-1 in 1968, so it wasn't like they had returned to their winning ways under Champion. As the opening days of training camp unfolded, I really thought I had a shot at making the team. I was only 26 years old and I thought I performed pretty well during the two weeks of two-a-days. Moreover, I made a couple of big plays in our final exhibition game, played in Calgary on a Sunday afternoon in early July. Even though we lost to the Stampeders 23-10, my performance caught the eye of *Vancouver Sun* columnist Denny Boyd. "Pokey Allen, the quiet veteran with the deep, penetrating eyes, the guy the newspapers have been saying might get dropped again for a rookie, had cut the credibility gap by hauling in a high, twisting Calgary punt and running it back to the Vancouver 45," he wrote following the game. I also had an interception that I returned from the B.C. eight-yard line to the Calgary 40.

Despite my two eye-catching plays I wasn't sure if I was going to make the cut. But I figured there was no sense in worrying about it, so some teammates and I decided to have a big blowout to celebrate the end of the exhibition season when we got back from Calgary that evening. (We didn't need much of an excuse to have a party.) At that time the sale of liquor on Sunday was illegal in British Columbia, but we weren't deterred. We called a bunch of friends and invited them to my place, a high-rise apartment overlooking English Bay. The players were definitely in a party mood because it was the end of the grueling preseason and they didn't have to practice the next day. When we started to run out of booze, we just called more people and told them to bring whatever they had. It turned into a pretty wild bash. Guys were hanging off the balcony, yelling at girls to come up and join us. It was like a scene out of *Animal House.*

It so happened that my sister and her husband (now her ex) had driven up from Seattle, about 140 miles away, to visit me; when they showed up I just told them to "join the party." Well, after several hours of revelry, the party was getting out of hand, so I thought it might be a good idea to leave—even though it was my place. "Let's get out of here," I said to Jennie and her husband around 1 a.m. "I think somebody is going to call the police and there's going to be all kinds of trouble." Well, I was right: As we were leaving the police were arriving. Needless to say, we didn't hang around; I went with Jennie and her husband to the hotel where they were staying while the cops came and shut down the party. I thought I was pretty clever evading the police, but the next day I got hit with a double whammy: I was evicted from my apartment and got cut by the Lions.

I WAS TERRIBLY disappointed by my failure to make the Lions, to say the least. Pro football was an excuse to stay young. I think everybody who has played football wants to continue playing it. For a while, it was difficult for me to come to grips with the fact that my playing career was really over. After I was released, I don't think I ever went to a Lions game. By the same token, I recognized that it was time to turn my attention to my coaching career. As for getting kicked out of my apartment, it was no big deal because I wanted to move to Burnaby anyway to be closer to the SFU campus. By the way, the Lions went 5-11 in 1969 and Champion was dismissed before the season ended.

I rejoined the football program at SFU, where I remained through 1976. We had a terrible year under Davies in 1969, going 1-6-1. Despite my professional woes during that time, my personal life took an interesting turn when I met a young woman, a fellow SFU employee who worked in the school's library. Her name was Tamara Pfefferle, and I found her very attractive. At the time, however, she was going out with Simon Fraser's top basketball player. We would run into each other on campus occasionally and engage in friendly chitchat, but that was about the extent of our interaction. Then one day she walked into my office and asked me out. I was hesitant because I knew she was dating this other guy. But she was so attractive, and I'm really weak when it comes to good-looking women. Anyway, she eventually stopped seeing the basketball player and we dated for more than a year.

Our relationship eventually grew serious, and in 1970 we got engaged. But the apprehension that has influenced virtually all of my romantic relationships—before and after I met Tammy—eventually crept into my head again. I was very attracted to Tammy and enjoyed being with her, but for some reason the thought of marriage began to frighten me; a few weeks before the holidays I told her I thought it would be better if we waited and broke off our engagement. When the semester break rolled around a week or so later she gave me back her engagement ring and left for Toronto to visit her sister while I went to spend Christmas with my folks in Missoula; the fate of our relationship was definitely up in the air. But after having some time to think about it, I guess Tammy decided she didn't like my decision to put off our wedding plans. During the holidays she called me at my parents' home from Toronto. "Pokey, I'm flying into Missoula. I've got my wedding dress," she announced. "If you don't want to marry me, we don't have to … but I want to."

Tammy arrived between Christmas and New Year's and stayed at my folks' house. From my perspective, it was an awkward situation. She wanted to get married and my parents concurred; I wasn't quite as enthusiastic. Still, Tammy and I went ahead and got the requisite blood tests for a marriage license a few days after Christmas. In addition to my cold feet, I also had to think about returning to work because I was due to hit the recruiting trail for SFU a few days after New Year's. And that helped me come up with the perfect excuse—or so I thought. I had my speech all set: "You know," I said to Tammy and my parents a day or two before New Year's, "as much as I'd like to get married, we can't. There's a two-day waiting period [by Montana law] after blood tests are taken before a wedding can be performed. There's bound to be a delay because of the holidays, and I have to leave soon after New Year's. We'll have to do it later … in Vancouver or something."

But my dad, the ex-cop, said he knew a judge who could expeditiously waive the rule and officiate a wedding ceremony. And, he added enthusiastically, *we could have the wedding right here in the living room before Tammy and I left for Vancouver!* So with little fanfare and even less forethought, in my opinion, it was decided we would get married on Saturday, January 2—just a day or two away.

If nothing else, it was a good reason to tie one on. On the evening of New Year's Day 1971, a Friday, Tammy and I headed to downtown Missoula with some friends of mine for an impromptu pre-wedding party. We hit various bars throughout the evening, and at around 2 a.m. Tammy wanted to go back to my folks' house and get some sleep. Most of the rest of our group stayed out dancing and drinking until about 4 a.m. I rolled in around 4:30 or 5.

Through the late morning and early afternoon of January 2, I sat in my parents' living room with Tammy and my folks, trying to lull away a hangover by watching the Gator Bowl on TV. Eventually, the judge showed up. I donned a suit jacket—I couldn't find a tie—and Tammy put on her wedding dress and we exchanged vows during halftime. Then we sat down and watched the rest of the game. The next morning we got in my car, drove to Seattle and stayed at the Edgewater Inn. That was our one-night honeymoon; the next day we were in British Columbia. I guess our marriage got off to a bad start our first day in Vancouver when I informed Tammy that we didn't have a place to live. I had moved out of my previous residence before the holidays, I explained, and hadn't really given much thought to finding another place. (But then I hadn't planned on returning with a wife either.) Anyway, I think we stayed in a hotel or something. The next day I was on the recruiting trail and Tammy went looking for a place for us to live.

In retrospect, I should have seen my little oversight as the precursor of a marriage that was destined to fail. I guess we just weren't compatible. She wanted a normal, come-home-from-work-and-have-dinner kind of marriage and I didn't want life to change. I was too much into going out and having fun and she was more of a homebody. I was messy, she was tidy. She wanted furniture, I didn't think chairs and lamps were all that necessary. After less than a year of marriage Tammy and I split up and eventually divorced. Despite our differences, our separation was amicable. Many years later, Tammy told a reporter, "Pokey was a great guy and lots of fun. He would have made a great brother; he just wasn't a very good husband." Tammy and I are still on good terms. She married Roger Kettlewell, a former B.C. teammate of mine who played defensive back for the Lions from 1966 through 1968; they live in the Vancouver area with their two kids.

After the wedding, I only saw my dad a few more times before he died. His health was going downhill fast. He had kidney disease, diabetes and heart problems and passed away in May 1971 while I was serving in the National Guard in Bellingham, Washington.

Even though I was living in Canada, I was still eligible for the military draft. My playing days and the first few years of my coaching career were at the height of the Vietnam War. And like a lot of young men at that time, I wasn't crazy about the idea of being shipped off to the other side of the globe to be shot at by an enemy I knew almost nothing about. My escape? I joined the Guard. I originally thought about trying to maintain my student deferment by enrolling in graduate school at Utah. Then I actually took a couple of graduate classes at the University of British Columbia, but I wasn't sure if or how long that would work. After my first year of pro ball, I looked into a National Guard Special Forces outfit based in Missoula. With the help of Marv Trask, my freshman football coach at Missoula High and a major in that detachment, I was able to join that unit for a six-year hitch.

During those six years I had to take Special Forces basic training in Utah and some other parts of the country and report to a military camp one weekend a month and two weeks each summer, but for the most part I was able to fulfill those obligations around my playing and coaching duties. When I got the preliminary military requirements out of the way, it was a matter of reporting to Fort Lewis in Washington state, and after that I ended up in a military police outfit in Bellingham, which was only a 75-minute drive from Vancouver.

I DON'T THINK coaching at a small school in Canada gave my career any kind of boost, but I liked working at Simon Fraser and I loved living in the Vancouver area. Nevertheless, some weird things happened with the football program during my nine seasons there. First of all, Lorne Davies, who was the school's athletic director in addition to being head football coach, made, in my opinion, some scheduling blunders that were a direct result of his religious beliefs. Davies was a member of the Church of God, a religion that believes the Sabbath is to be observed from sundown Friday to sundown Saturday. Now, I believe that religion is a very private matter, and I have no qualms with anyone's personal faith and how they carry out those beliefs. In no way do I mean to infer that Davies' faith was misguided. But in my opinion, his religious zeal in relation to his job as Simon Fraser's football coach went too far and not only hurt the program but jeopardized the well-being of our players during one eight-day span during the 1971 season.

By 1970 Simon Fraser had built a solid NAIA football program in the Pacific Northwest. In fact, we went 8-0 that year with wins over American schools such as Whitworth, Western Washington, Puget Sound and Portland State. In 1971 the coaching staff anticipated another banner year based on the fact that we had a large number of returning players. But then came our eight-day odyssey to Oregon. Because the Church of God's doctrine precluded Davies from working on Saturdays until dusk, he sought opponents who would agree to play the Clansmen at night. (And as everyone knows, almost all college football games are played on Saturday.) That led to a scheduling snafu that was inexcusable.

As expected, SFU routed its first three opponents—Pacific Univer-

sity, California Riverside and a semipro team from Everett, Washington—
by an average score of 45-5. Our fourth contest was originally supposed
to be against the Wolves of the Oregon College of Education (now Western Oregon State College) in Monmouth on Saturday, October 16, in a day
game. But when Southern Oregon State College informed Davies that it
was willing to host us on that date *in the evening,* Davies jumped at the
chance, figuring he could somehow drop the game with OCE. But when
the Wolves said no dice, Davies found himself with a big problem on his
hands. Davies and OCE eventually reached a compromise and agreed to
play on Monday, October 18, instead of the 16th. We made the trip to Oregon and won the first game, defeating Southern Oregon 22-14 in Ashland.
But then we had to turn around and play OCE in less than 48 hours and
got clobbered by the Wolves 38-0. To make matters worse, our starting
quarterback was injured in that contest.

Our problems didn't end there. We had another regularly scheduled
game at Portland State in just five days. We left Monmouth battered and
exhausted and returned by bus to British Columbia for a couple of days.
Later that week we reboarded the bus and drove down to Portland to face
the Vikings, who summarily beat us 21-3 on October 23. It was insane! We
were probably the only college football team in history to play three games
in eight days! Not only did Davies ruin what could have been another
great year, I think he placed our players in serious jeopardy by subjecting
them to such a brutal schedule. We finished the '71 season at 7-3.

In 1972 Davies continued his daft ways in regard to arranging SFU's
football games. This time he had a scheduling conflict because of his commitment to attend a religious conference that took him out of town for
several days in September of that year. The solution? To ensure that he
wouldn't miss any games, Davies didn't schedule the Clansmen's season
opener until September 30—a full three weeks into the season. By then
the school administration had seen enough of Davies' scheduling absur-
dities and asked him to step down as head coach after that first game; he
was replaced by defensive coordinator Tom Walker.

By that time I had moved up from DB coach to defensive coordinator and thought I had a shot at the head coaching job. I wasn't too upset
when Walker got the job, however, because he was Davies' heir apparent—a veteran coach who had been with the program since its inception
in 1965. I was only 29 and had been with the Clansmen program for four
seasons, probably too young and inexperienced in the eyes of Davies, who
was still the athletic director, and George Suart, SFU's vice president in

charge of athletics. Walker served as head coach for the final eight games of the '72 season and led the Clansmen to a 4-5 overall record.

It was around that time that I discovered rugby, which became quite a passion of mine for several years. Two of my teammates were Chris Beaton, another SFU assistant football coach whom I lived with, and Jerry Bradley, who had retired from pro football by then. Beaton, who is now SFU's head coach, and I would play with the Vancouver Meralomas Rugby Club in the spring, compete in tournaments in the summer, and coach football in the fall. One of the high points of our summers during that period was the annual Edmonton Rugbyfest. It was just a fantastic event and a lot of fun. I met a lot of good people during the years I played rugby and several of my longtime friends from Canada are former rugby players.

It was a fun time in my life, made all that more enjoyable by rugby and the social conviviality associated with it. Rugby and its inherent ruggedness had a real influence on me. It just seemed to go hand in hand with a lifestyle I could embrace. It seemed rugby players just had this attitude—play hard and party hard. My kind of sport.

In the spring of 1973 another odd development took place with the SFU football program. After less than one full season as head coach Walker resigned; naturally I once again sought the position, this time thinking I should get it. Unfortunately, I don't think I was Suart's kind of guy—too much of a free spirit, you might say. The other candidate was offensive coordinator Bob DeJulius, a family man. I, on the other hand, was divorced and too footloose and fancy-free.

You know, some people have a hard time understanding how people like me can get the job done and have fun at the same time. DeJulius was a good guy, but I didn't think he had what it took to be an effective head coach. I think Suart, whose official title was executive director of administration, realized that too. But it also seemed he didn't like the idea of me being in charge of the football program. "Pokey, we would name you head coach; you are obviously a good leader and everything," he said during my interview. "But you know, the only reason we can't give you the job outright is because you laugh and have too much fun."

I mean, talk about a warped outlook on life! "Whatever," I replied in exasperation when Suart was done explaining why he opposed my appointment as head coach. Instead he came up with a harebrained idea of co-head coaches. So for the next four seasons the Simon Fraser football program operated with DeJulius and me jointly sharing the head coaching duties. Despite the unusual arrangement, DeJulius and I got along fine and our football program continued to do well—to the point where some of the smaller schools we met on a regular basis began to grow weary of losing to us. For that reason we began to play larger schools such as Eastern Montana, Chico State, Nevada-Reno and Montana.

We only had 20 tuition scholarships but never had a losing season during the four years DeJulius and I shared the head coaching duties. We went 6-2 in 1973, 4-4 in '74, 5-4 in '75 and 5-5 in '76. In fact, we split our four games against Montana during my four-year stint as SFU's co-head coach.

Like I said, I enjoyed Vancouver immensely, but by the end of the 1976 season I had had my fill of what I thought was a nonsensical job situation and was ready to move on.

Chapter 7

An Able Assistant

Even though I grew up in Missoula, I never had a burning desire to play or coach for the University of Montana—that is until Grizzly head football coach Jack Swarthout stepped down after the 1975 season. I didn't exactly feel sudden pangs of homesickness when I heard about the job opening at UM, but I *did* see it as an opportunity to leave Simon Fraser. For three years I had put up with George Suart's decision to run the Clansmen football program with two head coaches—a total contrivance designed to avoid the problem rather than solve it —and had grown increasingly frustrated with the whole situation. I mean, what other college has appointed co-head coaches on a permanent basis? The idea was so lame that all it did was create needless complications; worst of all, it didn't appear SFU was in any big hurry to change the coaching arrangement anytime soon.

So when the Montana head coaching position opened up I submitted an application. I figured what the heck; I knew lots of people in Missoula, had eight years of coaching experience at the collegiate level, and was now 32 years old. But the school's powers that be decided to dip into Montana's prep ranks and select UM alumnus and Great Falls High coach Gene Carlson, who won a remarkable 77 percent of his games (108-32-8) and captured five Class AA state championships in his 15 years with the Bison. As a former Grizzly football and baseball standout in the late 1940s and early '50s, Carlson also had strong UM ties, which was something I couldn't put on my résumé despite the fact I was from Missoula.

So I remained at Simon Fraser as co-head coach for a fourth season, helping to guide the Clansmen to a 5-5 record in 1976. Our final game that year was a 45-17 loss to Carlson and the Grizzlies in Missoula; little did I know that it was to be my final game with SFU—played, ironically enough, in my hometown against the school that was to be my next employer.

With the win over SFU, Carlson finished his inaugural year at Montana with an unimpressive 4-6 record; it was the Grizzlies' fourth losing season in five years. At the conclusion of the '76 season Carlson was told by the UM administration to dismiss the coaches he had inherited from Swarthout and hire his own staff. Among the assistants Carlson had to let go was former Idaho and current Utah State head coach John L. Smith. Following word of Carlson's forced housecleaning, Ken Staninger, a close friend of mine and the color commentator for UM football radio broadcasts at the time, called and told me about the openings on the Montana football staff. Staninger, a Missoula native and active Grizzly booster, encouraged me to apply for the defensive coordinator position, adding he would put in a good word for me. But I was no stranger to Carlson; a number of years earlier I had played quarterback for Missoula County High against his Great Falls teams.

Prompted in part by Staninger's suggestion, I threw my hat in the ring yet again—marking my second application for a UM coaching position in as many years. This time I fared better as Carlson offered me the job as his defensive coordinator a few weeks later. Although I was anxious to leave the situation at Simon Fraser, I viewed a return to Missoula with a certain ambivalence. Vancouver, after all, was, and still is, one of the most vibrant and cosmopolitan cities in North America and had been my home for the better part of a decade. Plus, the thought of returning to the provincial setting of my youth gave me a certain backwoodsy feeling I wasn't all that excited about. Don't get me wrong; I didn't consider myself some city slicker who was too polished and worldly for a place like Missoula. It's just that I had outgrown my small-town roots and developed a taste and appreciation for the pleasures and advantages of living in a major city. "Allen is an urban animal," former Portland sports columnist Terry Frei wrote several years later. "The implications of his nickname to the contrary, he's not the type of guy for Laramie, Wyoming, or Manhattan, Kansas."

I was also concerned that my work as a UM assistant would be viewed with an inordinate amount of scrutiny because of my local ties. Perhaps if the Grizzly football program had been as successful back then as it is today, my decision would have been easier. But given the school's lackluster football history at the time, the prospect of helping Carlson turn the UM program into a winner seemed daunting at best. In both 1969 and '70 Swarthout led the Grizzlies to a 10-1 record and a berth in the Camellia Bowl. But those two years were the exception to more than three decades of gridiron mediocrity; even with the '69 and '70 seasons in the equation, Montana won only 37 percent of its games (114-188-2) between 1942 and 1975, and the school had only seven winning seasons—five under Swarthout—during that span.

It was during this period of deliberation that I began to realize my indecisiveness was starting to get the best of me; I needed a better way to handle stressful situations and not spend so much time agonizing over each and every decision. It didn't happen overnight, but I gradually developed a philosophy that has pretty much dictated my approach to life ever since: Make every experience an adventure. I believe this outlook has made difficult situations—such as my bout with cancer—easier for me to handle.

Steeled by my new outlook, I accepted Carlson's offer and moved to Missoula in the spring of 1977. For the first eight months I lived with Staninger—now a Missoula real estate businessman and sports agent and a local high school football star in his own right—until he got married in November of that year. Later I roomed with Grizzly basketball coach Mike Montgomery, who is now the head coach at Stanford.

Carlson was pretty straight-laced and conservative while I was quite the opposite, but we got along just fine and he treated me well. Years later a writer asked Gene why he had hired me when it was obvious that our personalities were so different. The answer was simple: He thought I could help him win. "I was well aware of Pokey's [playing and coaching] career after he played quarterback for Missoula against our Great Falls teams," Carlson said. "He was a fine high school athlete, and once he got into the coaching profession I considered him an outstanding coach and a first-rate recruiter. One reason I hired him was because I wanted a Montana flavor to our new coaching staff. I thought he would be an excellent defensive coordinator, and he was."

BY AND LARGE, I managed to enjoy my return to my hometown. Part of the reason was because I was near my mom and got to spend more time with her, as well as with old friends and classmates. Another reason was Kathy "Kate" Johnson, a local newscaster whom I started dating soon after I arrived in Missoula. Missoula television viewers knew her as Kathy Johnson, but Mike Montgomery and I decided that she should be called Kate within our circle of friends, and the name stuck. Kate and I first met when her station assigned her to interview some of the Grizzly assistant coaches for a story on the UM football program. Kate wasn't a sportscaster per se, but in a small television market like Missoula, most reporters are required to cover all aspects of the local news, including sports. Anyway, we started going out and went together for most of the three years I was with the UM football program.

During that time I bought a cabin on the west shore of Flathead Lake. Located just outside of Polson, Montana, about an hour and 15 minutes due north of Missoula, it has been my haven—my refuge from the stress and strain of the coaching profession and a place for friends to congregate—for nearly 20 years. Also during my first year as a UM assistant coach I befriended a Missoula restaurateur named Mike Munsey. Munsey and I had briefly met on a few occasions in the mid-70s, but when I started to frequent his establishment, a popular downtown steak house called The Depot, we soon became close friends. We were both single and in our mid-30s when we began to hang around together, playing golf and spending time at my place on Flathead Lake and at his cabin on nearby Swan Lake.

No matter where I was living or working, I would always make it back to Missoula for the holidays, and in the late '70s Mike and I began a tradition of spending part of Christmas Eve together at The Depot, often for a late-night dinner and a few glasses of champagne. I recall one December 24—I think it might have been the first year of our ritual—when we consumed more than just a few glasses of bubbly. Each Christmas Eve Mike would serve up an after-hours dinner in the restaurant for the employees who had worked the late shift that night. On this particular night before Christmas I showed up around midnight after spending the early portion of the night with my mother; when I arrived Mike broke out several bottles of Dom Perignon and his best champagne glasses. The champagne flowed freely for the next few hours and a few of Mike's employees stayed till 2 or 3 in the morning while Mike and I stayed up till 5 or 6, sitting in front of The Depot's fireplace, laughing, talking and toasting the new year. I'm sure we consumed a few hundred dollars worth of champagne that night.

We have continued our holiday custom through the years—a span of nearly two decades that has included seven different coaching jobs for me and marriage and parenthood for Mike. The one exception was in 1994 when I was diagnosed with cancer a few days before Christmas and had to remain in Boise for chemotherapy treatment. Nevertheless, I made it to Missoula and The Depot a few weeks later to belatedly celebrate the holidays with Munsey and his family and continue our tradition.

While living in Missoula, and later in Spokane, Washington, I continued my love affair with rugby, albeit to a lesser extent than when I resided in Canada and played for the Vancouver Meralomas Rugby Club. On more than one occasion Staninger, who played college football at Colorado State, and I would drive from Missoula to Edmonton—a round-trip of more than 1,200 miles—to meet Bradley and other players from the Meralomas and compete in the highly popular Edmonton Rugbyfest. From my perspective, the Edmonton tournament offered a double enticement: the rough-and-tumble competition on the field and the high-spirited socializing among the participants afterward. In my opinion, the Edmonton Rugbyfest was, and still is, what the sport is all about: a challenging athletic event and a rollicking social affair rolled into one. (I haven't been to the tournament for a long time, but I understand it's as popular and festive as ever.) Started in 1968, the Edmonton Rugbyfest is held each year during Canada's three-day Victoria Day weekend and typically draws between 30 and 50 teams from all over North America along with a few clubs from Europe. But unlike some of the more serious rugby tournaments, the light-hearted social activity associated with the Edmonton event is as big an attraction as the competition; I'd be lying if I said alcohol was not a major part of the scene when I was there. In fact, from my recollections most everyone in the tournament would play rugby and drink—some to the point of "chundering," which in rugby parlance means to vomit on the sidelines.

Despite the potentially volatile mix of alcohol consumption and contact sport, I never witnessed a fight in all the years I competed in the Edmonton Rugbyfest, which is pretty amazing given some players' overindulgence and the game's inherent violence. I mean, with 500-odd rugby players converging on one location, going to the same postgame keggers and barbecues, you would expect some bad blood to boil over at an occasional social gathering or two, but I never saw it. Most rugby matches are as intense and hard-hitting as anything that takes place on a football field, and the games in Edmonton were no exception. Rugby, however, prides itself as a sport that leaves the rough stuff on the field, and once the contest is over, the postgame revelry usually proceeds unabated.

Rugby was so much fun, in fact, that Staninger, Bradley and I started our own informal tournament in Polson in the late '70s. Aptly named the Flathead Falldown, we hosted it for three or four summers in a row. Although our tournament was small—one year we had just one match—it featured the same camaraderie among the participants as the Edmonton Rugbyfest; players from the Meralomas and the Edmonton Tigers along with other Canadian "ruggers" would make the trip to Montana, set up camp, play rugby during the day, and enjoy the festivities at night. At the height of its popularity, the Falldown drew about 200 people to its postgame gatherings. Just like the Edmonton Rugbyfest, the Flathead

Falldown's objective was twofold: play hard and party hard.

As much as I enjoyed rugby, age and injuries were beginning to take their toll. I suffered my most serious injury on a Saturday afternoon during my second or third spring with the UM football program. I had completed my coaching duties following a morning football practice session that day and went to watch a little rugby at a tournament hosted by the local rugby club, the Missoula Maggots. One team was a makeshift squad comprised primarily of former UM football players who hadn't played much rugby. The team that was scheduled to oppose the ex-Grizzlies was one player short, so I was asked if I wanted to fill in. It was a nice spring day, I was wearing shorts and had a pair of cleats in my car; I figured what the hell. I was handed a jersey and I joined in. During the match, I was running with the ball when I was upended by the ex-Grizzlies' Greg Anderson, a consensus All-America free safety for UM in the mid-70s. He knocked me right off my feet, and I landed on my wrist.

As I lay crumpled on the ground, players from both teams crowded around me, and in typical rugby fashion one of them finally asked, "You're still going to play, aren't you?" But I couldn't. I eventually got up, walked to my car and drove myself, one-handed, to the nearest emergency ward in Missoula. I had suffered a broken wrist and was in a cast for six weeks; for all practical purposes my days as a rugger were over. I participated in the Flathead Falldown another time or two and played in an "old boys tour" a year or so later, but that was the extent of it.

It was hardly the end of the good times, however; Bradley and I could always manufacture fun at Flathead Lake. Jerry and I eventually replaced the Flathead Falldown with an 18-event athletic competition we dubbed the "Amazing Relay." And now that rugby was no longer the sport of choice, the competition was also open to our female friends. Bradley, Staninger and I organized and officiated the event, which attracted dozens of friends and acquaintances the three summers we held it. The entrants were divided into men's and women's relay teams that competed in the various recreational activities available on or near Flathead Lake: running, canoeing, swimming, horseback riding, water basketball shooting, etc.—just about everything except hunting and fishing, both of which I hate. Even though we were no longer playing rugby, many members of the Tigers and Meralomas still made the trip from Canada to partake in the fun.

The Amazing Relay was a three-hour endurance test with rules that were ... well, loosely enforced and arbitrarily changed at the whims of the officials (Bradley and me), to make the competition close and the fin-

ish exciting. Case in point: While at the helm of the boat in the water-ski-
ing leg of the race, I would sometimes develop "engine problems" while
pulling the overall leaders. The boat would "inexplicably" slow down to
the point where the front-runners would sink into the lake, thus loosen-
ing their grip on first place. More than once Bradley and I were accused of
rigging certain parts of the relay. But of course two upstanding guys like
Jerry and me were beyond reproach; besides, we were running the show.
In the case of the skiers who wound up in the drink, I would sympatheti-
cally shrug my shoulders, plant tongue firmly in cheek and say, "Gee, I
don't understand ... the boat ran fine for all the others."

The penultimate leg of the Amazing Relay was a four-mile run to a
popular Polson watering hole called the Diamond Horseshoe Bar, where
the participants gathered for the final event: a beer chugalug. We planned
it so the final runner in both the men's and women's divisions crossed the
finish line and ran into the bar together. If one of the final racers was way
ahead, we'd pick up the trailing runner in a car and drop him or her off
near the finish line to make sure the pair ended the race at the same time.
Those two would culminate the Amazing Relay by downing a pitcher of
beer.

Like I said, Bradley and I had no trouble concocting fun at Flathead
Lake. After the Amazing Relay had run its course, I organized the Pokey
Allen Golf Invitational, and Bradley put together a boccie ball tournament.
After I took a coaching job with the University of California in 1982 Brad-
ley and I pretty much ended our organized sports events, but the cabin on
Flathead Lake has been a consistent and important part of my life—a gath-
ering place filled with family, friends and fun—for nearly two decades.
Without question, it has been the source of some of my fondest memories.
Bradley, Munsey, Staninger and many other friends and I have taught dozens of kids—including Jerry's two daughters, Tami and Kerri, my niece,
Tara Veazey, and nephew, Ryan Kirschling—to water ski on Flathead Lake.
I usually spend a good part of each July at the cabin, hosting a steady
stream of adult visitors and their kids. When the cabin is full of overnight
guests, it's a common practice to have the children flop in the nearby boat-
house. Many of those kids are adults now, and we're on the second generation of kids who come to Flathead Lake.

I have fond memories of almost all my times on Flathead Lake, but
there was one misadventure that wasn't much fun for three traveling companions and me. I had a new powerboat, a 19 and a half-foot Bayliner,
that I wanted to show off to my sister Jennie, her husband, Jack Kirschling,
and Diane Rees, my girlfriend at the time. I was still getting used to the

boat, so we thought a trip "up" the lake would be a fun way to try it out. Thirty miles long and five miles wide, Flathead Lake runs north and south and is the largest natural freshwater lake west of the Mississippi River. Since the cabin is situated on the lake's southwest end, a trip to the northeast shore and the Sitting Duck Saloon, our destination that evening, would be the longest distance a boat could traverse on Flathead Lake. Our foursome met Munsey for dinner at the Sitting Duck, and after an enjoyable meal and a few libations, Jennie, Jack, Diane and I got back on the boat around 11:30 p.m. for the 35-minute ride back to Polson.

The boat ran fine on the trip over, but it was just our luck to discover a few glitches in the system on the way back. First, the gas gauge was inaccurate; second, the fuel pump was all screwed up—and although I tried to explain that it wasn't my fault, my traveling companions were not very understanding when I informed them that we had run out of gas. Part of the reason for their displeasure was our location. If you were to mark an "X" at the spot where the lake's widest point met an imaginary line that was equal distance from the north and south shores, that's where we were—right smack in the middle. Needless to say, we were not a happy group that night. When the sun rose a few hours later, the irritation directed my way turned into resentment, then into icy stares as a cold front, which precluded any other boats from venturing our way, moved over the lake. We were cold and miserable and had no food and nowhere to go to the bathroom, except off the side of the boat. All morning long we drifted helplessly as the temperature dipped and the wind increased; swimming to shore was out of the question and the only thing that came close to a paddle was a fishing net I found under a seat. With the weather as it was, I honestly thought we were going to be stuck out there another night, but I didn't say anything; we were all uncomfortable and more than a little irritable as noon approached. To add to our misery, one member of our party (I won't say who) developed, um, gastrointestinal distress, making our plight even more unpleasant. Thank goodness a fishing boat finally came by around 2 p.m. and towed us in.

"Did you sleep?" Staninger asked me later. "Sleep?" I replied. "Are you kidding? I was afraid they were gonna commit mutiny and throw me overboard." I can laugh about it now, but those 14 hours adrift were pretty dreadful for all of us.

In addition to boating and other water sports, I was also doing some serious running during that period in my life. I initially got into the jogging craze in the late 1960s, and I can still remember thinking I was crazy the first time I ran more than a mile. Pretty soon, however, I was regularly running five to 10 miles at a time. I was pretty serious about it in the early and mid-70s and competed in several 10-kilometer races during that time. Then I *really* got serious and actually ran in two marathons, both in Vancouver. The first one was around 1978 and the other was in the early '80s. I trained to run in two or three other marathons after that but injured myself in the process. I was still running up to 40 miles a week until the early 1990s when my hips started bothering me; until I was diagnosed with cancer in late 1994 I was doing three-mile runs four or five times a week.

WHILE RUNNING, BOATING, playing rugby and hanging out with the likes of Staninger and Munsey was great fun, my coaching career hadn't exactly skyrocketed with the UM football program. As his record at Great Falls clearly showed, Carlson was a marvelous high school coach. But for whatever reason he couldn't work the same magic at Montana, and the program continued to flounder under his direction. We had a reasonably successful season in 1978, Carlson's third year and my second, grabbing a share of second place in the Big Sky Conference with a 4-2 league record and beating Boise State on the road 15-7. But we were 5-6 overall, and that year was sandwiched between records of 4-6 and 3-7 in 1977 and '79, respectively. The '79 season was especially frustrating; four losses—including a 37-35 setback to BSU—were by eight points or less. Despite the best efforts of Carlson and his staff, the Grizzlies sputtered to a 16-25 record—a winning clip of only 39 percent—during his four years at the helm.

There just didn't seem to be a commitment to winning at UM during that period, and the problem started with the facilities. The Grizzlies' dilapidated Dornblaser Stadium had all the charm of an abandoned warehouse—hardly the kind of facility to attract top recruits. We had some dedicated players such as Barry Sacks, a four-year letterman who started at linebacker his final two years; but in my opinion there were too many players of questionable character to make the program successful. Sacks, who coached for me at Portland State and is our current recruiting coordinator and defensive line coach at BSU, was the kind of hard-nosed and stand-up guy you want on your side. He was your typical overachiever—not very talented, not very big, but a kid who played hard; the kind of player you love to coach.

We could have used a few more players like Sacks in 1979; in our final game that year we lost to Portland State 40-32 as Viking quarterback Neil Lomax—who went on to star for the NFL's St. Louis/Phoenix Cardinals—riddled our defense, completing 30 of 48 passes for 361 yards and two TDs.

Our entire staff was fired by athletic director Harley Lewis after the season ended, and all the coaches, except for me, returned to the prep ranks. The following year Carlson wound up in Pasco, Washington, where he coached the local high school team through the mid-80s. Currently he is a vice principal at Pasco High and a couple of years away from retirement.

SO AFTER THREE seasons with the University of Montana I was out of work. It wasn't long, however, before I heard from another Big Sky coach—Weber State's Pete Riehlman, who was interested in hiring me as the Wildcats' quarterback coach. The job offer, especially the salary, sounded inviting, but I was wary of Riehlman, who was known as a difficult coach to work for. From 1968 through 1973 Riehlman had compiled a respectable 42-18 record as the head coach at Chico State. In 1974 he was hired as the offensive line coach for the Hawaii franchise of the World Football League; after the WFL folded in the fall of 1975 he served two years as a scout for a pro football combine before being hired by Weber State in 1977. Riehlman had an 11-21 record after three years at the Ogden, Utah, school, when he contacted me following the 1979 season. I think he was interested in hiring me for three primary reasons: First, as a defensive coordinator in the Big Sky I was already quite familiar with the other teams in the league; second, the defenses I devised against Weber State worked pretty well (UM held the Wildcats to 16 points in 1979 and just seven in 1978); third, I had been a successful college quarterback at nearby Utah, and I think he wanted to use my name to help promote his program.

Having coached against Riehlman at both Montana and Simon Fraser—the Clansmen beat Riehlman's Chico State Wildcats 21-13 in 1973, my first season as SFU co-head coach and his final year at the California school—I was vaguely familiar with his dubious reputation. But then, I wasn't in a position to be picky. Outside of a few postgame handshakes, Riehlman and I had never met, so I thought it best to form my own opinion and give him the benefit of the doubt. Besides, I needed a job, and the salary he quoted was more than I had made at UM. After talking on the phone, Riehlman and I agreed to meet at the 1980 NCAA football coaches' convention in New Orleans to discuss the job.

Since I wasn't in much of a position to negotiate, I was prepared to accept just about any offer Riehlman made. We met in New Orleans and he seemed nice enough. But while we were having a beer together, he said, "You know, you're going to have to shave off your moustache." I guess I didn't give it much thought at the time, but later, after I accepted his offer and returned to Missoula, I started to have second thoughts about my decision. I mean, for cryin' out loud, this was 1980! It's not like facial hair signified blatant nonconformity or subversive political views.

Still, I had made the commitment and was ready to move to Ogden a few weeks later. I didn't have a place to live, but Riehlman said he would set me up with a car and a room in the local Holiday Inn until I found a permanent residence. As it turned out, I wouldn't be needing any long-term accommodations.

As the time drew near for me to leave for my new job, I began to grow more concerned about Riehlman's reputation. I remember having dinner with Kate Johnson, whom I was still dating, a night or two before I was scheduled to leave. Over several glasses of wine, I began to list the pros and cons of my decision: Yes, I needed a job; no, Riehlman was said to be very dictatorial—hard on his players and especially hard on his assistants. Yes, I needed a job; no, I wasn't excited about living in Ogden. Yes, I needed a job; no, I really didn't want to work for Riehlman. Yes, I needed a job … My concerns notwithstanding, I knew my tenuous financial situation superseded my fear of Riehlman; I shaved my moustache and headed for Ogden a day or so later.

I flew into Salt Lake City while Riehlman was in California on a recruiting trip, so one of his assistant coaches picked me up at the airport. While we were waiting for my baggage we ran into another Weber State assistant who had just dropped off a couple of recruits. While my two new colleagues and I were talking, yet another assistant who was waiting to pick up some other recruits happened by. So here I was with three of my new co-workers, standing around in the airport terminal making small talk and joking, waiting for luggage to be unloaded and recruits to arrive. We were just shooting the breeze, getting to know each other; the conversation was lighthearted and humorous—that is until I popped the question: "Hey," I inquired amid the banter, "I've heard some bad stories about coach Riehlman. Are they true? Have you guys been treated badly?"

My questions brought an immediate halt to the laughter—followed by much foot-shuffling, throat-clearing and nervous looks among the three; suddenly they all looked like they had been beaten with a stick. After a solemn pause, one coach shook his head and said, "He expects us to be at his beck and call. I had to pick him up at 4:30 this morning to drive him [some 30 miles] to the airport." I said, "Oh shit, you're kidding, aren't you?" But he wasn't. Then another coach said, "Don't worry about it, the quarterback coach is usually treated a lot better than the rest of us."

But that didn't help. Now I *really* started having seconds thoughts about working for Riehlman. When my baggage finally showed up, I followed the coach who had met me at the gate out to the parking lot and to the car Riehlman had arranged for me to use. "Don't forget, you have a press conference tomorrow morning at 9," the coach said before we parted. "Riehlman won't be there. Just drive to the school and the athletic director [Gary Crompton] will introduce you to the media; be prepared to answer some questions."

Well, shoot , as I drove to the motel, my mind was awash with misgivings and apprehension; I didn't sleep at all that night. I knew I would make more money at Weber than I had at Montana, but I just didn't have a good feeling about Riehlman. After staying up in my room all night, I decided I just couldn't do it. At 7 a.m. I called Crompton on the phone. "I have some personal business and I can't take this job," I said. "I have some problems. I'm driving to the airport. I have a flight out of here. I'll leave the keys to the car at the Northwest counter. Sorry."

And that was it. I was outta there, back to Montana. It had to be the shortest coaching stint in the history of NCAA football. I figure I was employed by Weber State for about 16 hours. My ill-advised trip to Ogden turned out to be a bigger fiasco than my brief flight from the Utah football program almost 20 years earlier. (I know, I know. ... What about this newfound philosophy about making everything an adventure? Well, all I can say is this was one adventure I didn't want to go on.)

If I didn't have a reputation as a flake then, I sure did after that episode. Looking back, I think I made the right choice. Riehlman went 4-7 in 1980, his fourth losing season in as many years at Weber State, and got canned after a 75-0 season-ending loss to Portland State. His overall record with the Wildcats was 15-28. Funny thing, most fellow coaches applauded my decision because Riehlman was widely regarded as a—I'll be kind here—genuinely unpopular fellow. The last I heard, he was out of football and living somewhere in California.

SO I WAS back in Missoula and out of a job. In my effort to attain gainful employment, I contacted Eastern Washington head coach Dick Zornes, whom I knew from my days in Canada (he was the defensive back coach with the B.C. Lions when I was coaching at Simon Fraser). "Sure, I'll give you a job," Zornes said, "but I can't give you a full-time position until the fall; I can give you $5,000 for the recruiting season and spring ball." That was all I needed to hear; in a matter of days I was on my way to the Cheney, Washington, school. I eventually found a place to live in Spokane and joined Zornes' staff, taking over as defensive coordinator by the start of the 1980 season. One nice aspect to my job with EWU was the school's relative proximity to Flathead Lake (approximately 200 miles) and Vancouver (around 400 miles). By remaining in the Pacific Northwest, I was still able to visit Bradley and other friends in Canada and my mom in Missoula, and continue the Flathead Falldown for a couple more years. After I moved to Spokane, Kate Johnson and I broke up. (She later left the Missoula TV station and went to work for an advertising agency in Billings. Today Kate Johnson Hart lives with her husband and three kids in Spokane.) I dated a woman named Patsy McNamara after that, and in 1981 a woman named Kim Williams and I began a relationship that lasted about four years, which is a long time for me.

In 1980, Zornes' second year, the Eagles went 6-4; two of those losses were to Montana and Simon Fraser. In 1981 EWU posted a 7-3 record. With the exception of a season-opening 34-10 road loss to Idaho State, which went on to win the Division I-AA national championship that year, we were in every game and conceivably could have gone 9-1. I don't like to toot my own horn, but I think I was starting to be recognized as a pretty talented defensive coach.

Part of the reason was the performance of Eastern Washington's defensive unit in 1981. With the exception of the ISU loss, we gave up no more than 14 points that year. Our defense had three shutouts and gave up an average of less than 10 points per game. I certainly can't take all the credit for the Eagles' outstanding defensive performance in '81; among the other assistants was first-year linebacker coach Tom Mason, who would become a close friend and one of my top assistants at Portland State and Boise State. (Mason served as the Broncos' interim head coach for all but the final two games of the 1996 season while I was in British Columbia on medical leave seeking alternative cancer treatment.) Zornes coached at EWU for 15 seasons, posting an 89-66-2 record. He stepped down to take an assistant athletic director's position at the school after the 1993 season.

After two years at EWU, I got my first opportunity to coach in a big-time college football program with Joe Kapp at the University of California. My eventual move to Berkeley actually began in 1979 when I was still with the Montana football program. My recruiting duties for the Grizzlies included occasional trips to the Seattle area; while in that neck of the woods I would occasionally drive up to Vancouver and visit Bradley and some other friends. On a couple of those trips, I ran into Kapp, my former teammate with the B.C. Lions who by then had retired from the NFL. Kapp, who at the time had no coaching experience, told me that California coach Roger Theder was going to lose his job and that he, Kapp, was going to be named the Golden Bears' new coach. "When?" I asked Kapp. "Soon," he replied. "And I want to hire you as an assistant." But I didn't believe him; given his inexperience, I just couldn't imagine Joe getting the job as the head coach at a Pac-10 school.

In 1979 Theder's job seemed secure. He led the Bears to a respectable 7-5 record and a berth in the Garden State Bowl. But in 1980 it appeared the Cal coach's dismissal was imminent as his team went into its season finale against Stanford with a 2-8 record. But the Bears managed to beat the Cardinal 28-23, which, according to Kapp, allowed Theder to keep his job for another year.

As it turned out, Kapp knew what he was talking about. In 1981 Cal finished with a 2-9 record, Theder was axed and Kapp, who was an All-America quarterback for the Bears and led them to the 1959 Rose Bowl, was named the school's new head coach. I was astonished, but I guess I shouldn't have been. Kapp was nothing if not a masterful self-promoter. I think he got the Cal job by dint of charisma, connections with the school, and his ability to influence and impress Cal athletic director Dave Maggard. There was no denying that Kapp had a certain magnetism, which was especially evident in 1969 when he led the Minnesota Vikings to Super Bowl IV. But there is more to coaching than celebrity status and a strong personality. Strong personality? Make that stubborn—a characteristic of Kapp's that nearly brought us to blows more than once.

True to his word, one of the first things Kapp did was hire me as his defensive back coach. I certainly don't regret my decision to join Kapp, but I must say that 1982, my one and only year at Cal, was one of the most bizarre football seasons of my life—culminated by perhaps the most bizarre game-ending play in college football history. But then, this was Berkeley, where the unusual is commonplace.

One obvious problem stemmed from Kapp's decision to name a bunch of his old cronies and former teammates to his staff. While Joe had enough sense to hire a few veteran coaches such as Ron Lynn (16 years in the business), Lary Kuharich (12 years) and me (14), the majority of our staff—most notably Kapp himself—had little or no college coaching experience. Bill Cooper, a college teammate of Kapp's, had some limited experience, but most of the other assistants were green. Sam Gruneisen and Charlie West, who played with Kapp on the Vikings, went on to coach in the NFL, but at the time they were untested.

Another member of Kapp's staff that season was a first-year graduate assistant named Al Borges, who moved to the collegiate level for the first time after seven years as an assistant in California's high school ranks. Borges later became my offensive coordinator at both Portland State and

Boise State. Even though he was new to the ways of coaching football at the collegiate level, it was evident that Al had a great offensive mind, a talent that would bring us both a great deal of success a few years down the road. After working for me from 1986 through 1994 Al left our staff at BSU in 1995 to become offensive coordinator at the University of Oregon; in '96 he took over as offensive coordinator at UCLA.

I didn't realize how much I knew about football until I started comparing myself to Kapp. I mean, he had some really off-the-wall concepts about the game. Problem was I always had to be the one to tell him when he was off his rocker. Whenever Joe came up with one of his goofy ideas, sometimes right in the middle of a game, the other coaches would say, "Pokey, Joe will listen to you. You gotta go talk him out of it." Then I would have to go to Kapp and say something like, "Joe, we can't do this," to which he would reply something like, "What the fuck do you mean we can't do this!?" And a shouting match would usually ensue.

Kapp pulled all kinds of weird stuff that year in Berkeley. One example took place in our season opener at Colorado—Kapp's coaching debut and my first game as a Division I coach. We built a 21-3 lead early in the third quarter, and Kapp (prematurely) decided to send in the substitutes. Colorado proceeded to score two touchdowns before the quarter was over and all of a sudden our lead was cut to 24-17 going into the final period. Kapp reinserted our starters, but by then Colorado had the momentum.

Our defense was able to hold the Buffaloes at bay throughout the fourth quarter and we had the ball and a 24-17 lead with about a minute and a half remaining. I was on the sidelines talking on my headset to Lynn, who was in the press box. "We've got it won, Ron," I remember saying. "I'll see you downstairs." Then I looked over at Kapp who was huddling with our offensive coaches. "What the hell is he doing?" I said into my microphone to Lynn. "We don't need to confer; we're in our victory formation." But instead of calling a couple of running plays and milking the clock, Kapp was about to instruct Gale Gilbert, our sophomore quarterback, to throw the ball! I took off my headset, trotted over to Kapp and said, "Joe, what are you doing?" "They can't cover the post," Kapp answered. I couldn't believe it! "God, no, don't!" I begged. "Just have Gilbert take a knee."

"Fuck you!" he replied. "I'm the fuckin' head coach and we're going to score one more touchdown." So on second down in our own territory Gilbert dropped back to pass; we all damn near died when his throw was tipped at the line of scrimmage. Fortunately, the ball fell to the ground, but the incompletion stopped the clock (the last thing we wanted to happen), with about a minute remaining. Now it was third down and we couldn't run out the clock anymore. Now Kapp looked at me and asked, "What should I do?" I said, "Joe, I'd run the ball and then we're going to have to punt and hope they don't complete a long pass." "Fuck you!" he shouted, as if it was my fault we were in this predicament. But Kapp did what I suggested, and after one run we punted the ball to Colorado. We could have run out the clock, but instead the Buffaloes got the ball back, albeit deep in their own territory, with 40 seconds remaining and a chance to tie the game. Fortunately, defensive back Richard Rodgers intercepted a pass by Colorado quarterback Randy Essington in the closing seconds and returned it 34 yards for a game-clinching touchdown. But our 31-17 win was much closer, and more nerve-racking, than it needed to be.

Another time we were having a last-minute coaches' meeting before a game and Kapp announced, "You know what I'd like to do? I'd like to have the team form a 'C' when we go out on the field for our pregame warm-up." Nobody said a word, so Kapp said, "OK, that's what we'll do. Now let's get out of here!" But before our perplexed staff shuffled out of Kapp's office, I had to once again work up the courage to challenge our boss' logic. "Uh, Joe, how are we going to do that?" I asked. "We've got to practice something like that. You can't just tell a football team five minutes before it's supposed to go out on a football field to form a 'C.'"

My entreaties with Kapp worked at times, but they were never easy. Our coaches' meetings were regularly disrupted by a shouting match between Kapp and me. I mean, he was one of the most headstrong people I have ever met, and he definitely didn't like his authority challenged. We were at each other's throats all season. It was just crazy. Although I respected Kapp for his leadership qualities, working for Joe was just too much of a drain. I think if he had mellowed, used some common sense, and gained some technical experience he could have been an outstanding coach. But the sheer force of a coach's will alone won't win a lot of games, and in 1982 he simply didn't have the experience.

Not all of the strange things that happened to me during my year at Cal took place on the football field. One time I found myself naked in an Everett, Washington, hotel lobby while on a recruiting trip for the Bears. Before I relate this story, I should preface it by admitting that I'm a somnambulist—a sleepwalker. After spending a week in the Pacific Northwest on the recruiting trail, I decided to stay in Everett and meet Kim Williams, whom I had been dating for about a year, for a weekend of, um, fun and relaxation. Kim flew over from Spokane and we stayed in a hotel that was part of the chain she was working for at the time. On that first night we went out and had dinner—drinking, dancing, laughing and having a great time. Now, If I'm in a strange place and I've been drinking, I've got to be really careful because of my tendency to sleepwalk. Anyway, sometime in the middle of the night, it must have been about 3 or 4 a.m., I got out of bed. I was either sleepwalking or looking for the bathroom or both. But instead of going into the bathroom, I opened the other door in the room and groggily stepped into the hallway. The bright lights and the click of the door behind me woke me up instantly. It only took me a second to realize what I had done—and that I was in my birthday suit.

I immediately knocked on the door with little taps so as not to wake any other guests. "Kim … Kim," I pleaded in a half-whisper. "Let me in." But Kim was passed out, so I began knocking, then pounding, on the door to no avail. I must have pounded too hard because a couple of other doors began to open. "Oh, shit," I gasped as I dashed down the hall. "This isn't working."

I pulled some drapes off a hallway window and wrapped them around me. I wasn't feeling real good from all the drinking I had done and started looking around for a place to sleep it off. But I couldn't find anywhere to hide, and after about 90 minutes wandering the halls dressed like the Sheik of Araby I finally went down to the lobby. I thought about throwing myself on the mercy of the front desk and just telling them what had happened. But when I tiptoed into the lobby at around 5 a.m. there was no one behind the desk. "Jesus! What am I gonna do now?" I muttered to myself. That's when I saw the pay phones. I grabbed a phone, called the operator, placed a collect call to our room, woke up Kim, told her to open the door, ran up three flights of stairs, made a mad dash down the hallway and into the room. "I'll tell you later," I said to Kim. "I'm going back to bed."

LIKE I SAID, my year with the Cal football program was strange indeed; our season-opening win over Colorado was indicative of the strangeness. Three of our losses were annihilations—50-7 to Washington, 42-0 to Southern Cal and 47-31 to UCLA—while our fourth defeat was a 15-0 setback at the hands of Arizona State. Our defense played well and limited the Sun Devils to one TD, but our offense struggled the entire game and crossed the 50-yard line just once the entire second half. Despite those rather lopsided affairs, we ended up going 7-4 and Kapp was named Pac-10 Coach of the Year.

No question about it, though, the highlight of my year at Cal was

The Play, one of the most incredible finishes in college football history. We were at home in our season finale against archrival Stanford and John Elway, who was playing in his last collegiate game. Elway, it goes without saying, is one of the best quarterbacks ever to play the game; he was just as formidable in college back then as he is in the pros today. We knew our only chance against Elway was for our defensive unit to take some risks and apply as much pressure on him as we could. As the game started, I took my place on the sidelines, adjusted my headset and hoped for the best. "Well, here goes," I murmured into the microphone to Lynn, who was up in the press box at the other end of our hookup. Lynn—who went on to serve as defensive coordinator for the USFL's Oakland Invaders and the NFL's San Diego Chargers, Cincinnati Bengals and Washington Redskins—said nothing in reply. I think he was too worried about what Elway could do to our team if he got on a roll.

Our strategy worked well throughout the first half as our defense kept Elway off balance with a variety of alignments mixed with an all-out blitz to keep him on his toes. Meanwhile, Gilbert was doing an efficient job, leading the Bears to a 10-0 halftime lead. But in the second half Elway adjusted to our stunts and rallied the Cardinal to a pair of third-quarter touchdowns and a 14-10 lead. Cal regained the lead early in the fourth quarter on a 35-yard field goal by Joe Cooper and a 32-yard TD pass from Gilbert to Wes Howell. We failed on our two-point conversion attempt following Howell's score, but still clung to a 19-14 lead. Stanford's Mark Harmon later kicked a 22-yard field goal to cut the lead to 19-17 with five and a half minutes remaining in the game.

With 1:27 remaining we had to punt, giving Elway the ball deep in his own territory. After three unsuccessful plays, Elway and the Cardinal offense found themselves in a fourth-and-17 situation at their own 13. The next play, however, was vintage John Elway. We threw a blitz at the Cardinal offense and appeared to have Elway trapped. "We got him! We got him!" Lynn screamed from the press box into my headset. But Elway threaded a 29-yard pass to wide receiver Emile Harry for a first down at the Stanford 42; one of our linebackers could have knocked the ball down, but he couldn't react in time because it had been thrown so hard.

It's hard to explain, but the ball actually makes a whistling sound when Elway is throwing hard, and he was firing bullets now. During that final drive, even with the crowd going wild, I could actually hear a different sound from the ball—a higher-pitched whir-whir-whir of its laces—as it left Elway's hand and zipped through the air before hitting the receiver's hands with a loud slap. The speed and accuracy of his throws were something to behold as he quickly and efficiently moved the Cardinal offense down the field. Throughout his storied career, Elway's trademark has been his ability to rally his team to victory in the closing moments; it looked like we were about to become yet another victim of one of those patented comebacks. Elway maneuvered the Cardinal into field goal range, and with four seconds left Harmon kicked a 35-yarder for what appeared to be a 20-19 victory and a spectacular finish to Elway's collegiate career.

The Stanford-Cal rivalry is as intense as any in college football, which made our apparent loss all that much more bitter. The Cardinal players and their fans were going crazy. The place was almost out of control. Stanford was given an unsportsmanlike conduct penalty for celebrating on the field too excessively after Harmon's field goal, but Elway and his teammates didn't care. Our team was totally dejected; we thought we had lost the game. I glanced over at Kapp, who stared at the ground in dismay. Charlie West was crestfallen and the rest of the players and coaches stood in silence. Behind me, as our return team was preparing to take the field for the game's final play, I heard some of the players say, "Hey, play the return like rugby—lateral, lateral, lateral—and see what we can do."

It was still total confusion as we lined up for the final play. In fact, we had just 10 players on the field for the kickoff. With a 15-yard penalty assessed on the kickoff, Stanford had to kick from its own 25, but it seemed like a mere formality. Harmon booted a squib kick that sailed to the Cal return team's left and was gathered in by Kevin Moen at the Bear 43.

Then it happened. Moen headed right and lateraled to special teams captain Richard Rodgers near midfield. Rodgers carried the ball briefly and pitched it to Dwight Garner. Garner was hit by three or four Stanford players, but just before they all hit the ground, Garner somehow managed to get rid of the ball, which seemed to squirt out of the pile of players and back into Rodgers' hands. Now it was really getting confusing because nearly everyone in the stadium thought the game was over; Stanford's bench had emptied onto the field, and so had both marching bands, from each end zone. Rodgers was now racing along the right sideline in Stanford territory. As a Cardinal defender moved in to stop him, Rodgers flipped the ball to Mariet Ford near the Stanford 45. Now Stanford players *and* band members were in the way. At the Cardinal 25-yard line Ford tossed a no-look lateral to Moen and wiped out two Stanford defenders. Moen got a block from Howell, sprinted through the Stanford band, bowled over a trumpet player and ran into the end zone.

Everybody was stunned, but there were penalty flags on the field. I was watching the referee, who was running through the crowd trying to locate his fellow officials to find out what the flags were for and if there was any reason why the play shouldn't stand. Players, band members and hundreds of people were milling around on the field. After a brief huddle, the officials ruled that the penalty was against Stanford for too many players on the field and that the touchdown was good. The place went crazy! Cal's cannon, which is fired after each score, went off. It was total bedlam—the most amazing thing I had ever seen on a football field! Cal had stunned Stanford 25-20!

It was a wild and raucous scene in our locker room, where I remained for an hour and a half, and when I came out, there were *still* thousands of wildly cheering people in the stands. It was total pandemonium outside Memorial Stadium, a scene that must have been what V-J Day looked like. Revelers flooded Bancroft Avenue, dancing and celebrating as Kapp and I drove to a postgame celebration at the Marriott Hotel in Berkeley. Normally, it takes 10 to 15 minutes to drive from the stadium to the Marriott, but this time it took us about an hour and a half. We were driving by all the sororities and fraternities; people were handing us beers and drinks through the car window and the band was still playing up and down the street. Our incredible win over Stanford that November afternoon in 1982 sparked the wildest and longest celebration I have ever seen.

Kapp remained as Cal's head coach through the 1986 season. Today he is a businessman in the San Jose area. I am told one of his current ventures is a new pro football league. Like I said, Kapp was a born leader, but I decided one year as an assistant under Joe was enough. My next stop was the pros.

Chapter 8

USFL Years

C oaching has been my life, but it hasn't been my sole source of income. In the late 1970s and early '80s I joined a group of friends from Canada and the U.S. who invested in gold and oil stocks that performed quite well. I was able to parlay those profits into some other investments, and at one point in my life I guess you could say I was kind of wealthy, albeit briefly.

In the late '70s our group hit a real runner with a stock called Lincoln Resources. Basically, the stock went from 25 cents to $18 a share. During that time I had read a book on rental properties, and decided to invest a portion of my stock earnings in some property. I bought four houses in Missoula, which I rented out, and 20 acres of land, which I subdivided. It seemed like in a matter of weeks I had amassed a considerable amount of money. When I joined the football program at Eastern Washington in the spring of 1980, I was able to buy a fairly upscale house in Spokane.

During our hot streak our group of investors switched all the funds we had in Lincoln Resources to two oil stocks in Texas, both of which took off. For a brief time, we were rolling in the dough. We were all bachelors between 33 and 40 who fancied ourselves as some high-rolling playboys. One spring during our period of good fortune we flew into Sun Valley in a private plane to do some skiing and catch singer/songwriter Jerry Jeff Walker in concert. I remember one day in particular. I skied one of the big mountains in Sun Valley and when I got to the bottom of the hill I called my broker, who told me our stock would be up another 25 cents that day, so I told him to buy another 10,000 shares. By the end of the day, I thought I was a millionaire. With all my investments combined, I think I was pretty close to the seven-figure mark. But it was all on paper.

When my buddies and I went to listen to Walker perform in a Sun Valley bar a day or so later we ended up sitting with several women and a few other people. Feeling pretty good about my financial situation and enjoying the show, I decided to celebrate and bought a double round of kamikazes for our table. I pulled out a credit card, figuring what the hell, I can afford it. I guess I didn't realize how many people were in our party because the bill for that one round was something like $500. I'll never forget that because a few months later I could hardly afford to buy myself a beer.

The sluggish economy of the early 1980s was the reason for my financial downturn. The stock market hit the skids and so did the real estate market. I couldn't sell my stock interests and I couldn't rent or sell my houses. When I left Eastern Washington for my job at Cal I gave my house in Spokane back to the mortgage company because I couldn't find a buyer. It was a beautiful house that I hated to give up, but I had no choice.

Truth be told, I was out of my league with my fellow investors. I mean, most of these guys, including Jerry Bradley, were—and still are in some cases—high rollers who would think nothing of being $10 million up or $10 million down; it's a way of life for them. I still dabble in stocks a little today, but the stakes are nowhere near as high as they used to be.

DESPITE MY INTEREST in stocks and real estate, my first love has always been coaching. And the events surrounding that chaotic scene in and around the University of California's Memorial Stadium following the Golden Bears' incredible win over Stanford that autumn afternoon in 1982 seemed to epitomize my career to that point. From Burnaby to Missoula, to a one-night stand in Ogden, to Cheney and Berkeley, it had been a 15-year odyssey—unusual at times and unpredictable on occasion with more strange and interesting twists and turns still to come.

On a personal note, Kim Williams and I lived together during my year at Cal and she also joined me for the first several months I worked for the L.A. Express of the United States Football League. But we split up in Los Angeles and she eventually moved back to Spokane. All told, our relationship lasted about four years. Kim, whose name is now Kim Nance, is married and lives in Seattle.

When I joined the Simon Fraser staff in the summer of 1968 I was a 25-year-old rookie coach with an uncertain future. Now, here I was in late 1982, a reputable veteran, two months short of my 40th birthday—still unsure of where my football fortunes would take me. I had, however, come to one conclusion: I wanted to coach in the National Football League. That, along with Kapp's maddening coaching style, is what compelled me to leave Cal after the 1982 season for an assistant coach's position with the Express of the fledgling USFL. How could a job in a league that had yet to play a game help me reach the NFL? In my mind, the answer was simple: L.A. head coach Hugh Campbell. The formula went like this: impressive, successful head coach + national exposure = NFL coaching jobs for the aforementioned coach and his loyal staff.

I thought if I played my cards right, Campbell would become an instant winner in the USFL (just as he had done in the Canadian Football League), land a job as an NFL head coach, and take me along with him—a premise that would prove to be half right a year later.

Given Campbell's unprecedented success with the CFL's Edmonton Eskimos from 1977 through 1982—five consecutive Grey Cups and six divisional titles in as many years—and the USFL's TV package with ABC and ESPN, the scenario I envisioned seemed perfectly plausible. Although Campbell's name was occasionally bandied about when an NFL head coaching position opened up in the early '80s, for the most part he was an unknown in the U.S. But now he had escaped the anonymity of the Canadian league and would be coaching in front of a national television audience in the States. Bolstered by its TV packages, the signing of several high-profile players, and the deep pockets of owners such as developer Donald Trump, the upstart USFL planned to give the mighty NFL a run for its money as it prepared for its inaugural season in 1983.

The inception of a second pro football league was nothing new, but such undertakings have rarely put a dent in the NFL's armor of prosperity. While the Canadian Football League posed no real threat to the NFL and the Continental Football League and similar ventures have come and gone, the American Football League proved to be the exception. Throughout most of the 1960s the AFL became a legitimate rival, challenging the NFL for television dollars and engaging in salary wars for the nation's top collegiate players. When the two leagues merged in 1970 the NFL's power and popularity increased even more, giving subsequent upstarts, such as the World Football League, even less of a chance of survival. Started in 1974, the WFL barely lasted two years.

Despite the WFL's failure a decade earlier, the USFL had high expectations in its attempt to compete with the NFL. The league had been able to lure some big-name head coaches—George Allen (Chicago), Chuck Fairbanks (New Jersey), Red Miller (Denver) and John Ralston (Oakland)—into the fold, and it gained further credibility when it signed several of the nation's top college prospects, including 1982 Heisman Trophy winner Herschel Walker. Walker, who signed a multimillion dollar deal with Trump's New Jersey Generals instead of returning to the University of Georgia for his final year, was the USFL's big drawing card in 1983, but he was just one player among many the USFL landed that first year. The Philadelphia Stars signed three standouts—North Carolina running back Kelvin Bryant, UCLA offensive tackle Irv Eatman and BYU center Bart Oates—who were projected to go in the early rounds of the NFL draft while the Michigan Panthers came to terms with University of Michigan wide receiver Anthony Carter and Northwestern Louisiana State quarterback Bobby Hebert.

There was also a handful of familiar names joining the USFL thanks in part to Allen. Known for his quick-fix approach of acquiring older players in an attempt to produce immediate results, the Chicago Blitz coach continued that practice in the new league, signing NFL veterans such as quarterback Greg Landry, linebacker Stan White, cornerback Virgil Livers, and defensive linemen Coy Bacon and Joe Ehrmann. Allen planned to merge their considerable experience with talented rookies such as Grambling wide receiver Trumaine Johnson and Ohio State running back Tim Spencer, making Chicago was one of the preseason favorites.

With the possible exception of the UCLA passing duo of quarterback Tom Ramsey and wide receiver Jojo Townsell, the Express' roster was comprised of no-name players in 1983. Still, Campbell had worked wonders in the CFL and I was certain we could do the same in the USFL. It would only be a matter of time, I believed, before the NFL would beckon.

Campbell and I crossed paths more than once before I joined his staff. We played against each other in the CFL in the mid-60s and were coaching rivals in the college ranks once after that. Hugh was a standout wide receiver for the Saskatchewan Roughriders from 1963 through 1969—he skipped the '68 season to work as an assistant coach at Washington State, his alma mater—and earned all-star honors in 1965 and 1966, the two seasons I started in British Columbia's defensive backfield (coincidence, I'm sure). Before he joined the CFL coaching ranks, Campbell was the opposing head coach at Whitworth College in Spokane during the 1975 season when I was co-head coach at Simon Fraser. We beat Campbell's Pirates 27-7 that year. Despite Campbell's familiarity with me, it was actually Steve Shafer, a former B.C. Lions teammate of mine and the Express' defensive coordinator, who convinced Campbell to hire me as the team's defensive line coach in January of 1983. Another assistant hired by the Express that year was Keith Gilbertson, who would later become the head coach at Idaho and California before joining the NFL's Seattle Seahawks as an assistant in 1996.

If all went well, the 12-team USFL planned to eventually compete head-to-head with the NFL. But the new league's owners thought it best to play it safe at the outset, adopting an 18-game "spring" schedule—a slate of games that would begin in early March and culminate with the league championship in mid-July. The flaw in that plan, however, was the limited time frame between the conclusion of the traditional 1982 season, the USFL's draft in early January, and the start of the league's season on March 6. With most coaches coming to the USFL from other pro teams or college programs—jobs they were committed to through the end of the '82 season—many of the league's coaching staffs were slow to come together. The Express was no exception. Starting from ground zero, we had a mere five weeks to assemble our team.

Like the rest of the league, we had a difficult task at hand, but Mother Nature was especially unkind to our team that spring. Southern California is one of the most arid regions in North America, but in the early weeks of 1983 it rained for days on end, or so it seemed. Because the Los Angeles area is poorly prepared to handle an excessive amount of precipitation, the wet conditions wreaked havoc with the free-agent tryout camps we held at various high school football fields throughout the L.A. area; with inadequate drainage systems and hundreds of prospects ripping up the soft turf, the fields we used quickly turned into quagmires. The conditions were terrible during those wet weeks; we tore apart one field and moved on to the next a day or so later.

It was a real zoo putting a new team together in such a short time, and the pressure seemed to be getting to Campbell. I'll never forget when we had a weekend tryout camp with about 1,000 aspirants. I had just been with the Express for a week, still trying to get paperwork done, my office organized and duties straight. We were on the field conducting drills; I had just run about 14 prospects through an initial agility drill when Campbell walked up and said, "OK, give me your evaluation."

"Hugh, that was our first drill," I explained. "I can't tell you anything yet." Well, he jumped all over me. I couldn't believe it because he was usually such a soft-spoken guy. "Pokey!" he yelled. "I'm going to the next group, and you better have some answers for me when I get back!" It was the weirdest thing, so unlike him. Later, when I mentioned his little tirade, he said he didn't even remember it. I have no idea why he did it. I mean, talk about a laissez-faire coach, he was it. Then things got even more stressful a few weeks later when Shafer resigned to join the Los Angeles Rams as their defensive back coach. (Currently, Steve, a close friend of mine, is the Oakland Raiders' DB coach.) With Shafer's departure, I became the Express' defensive coordinator, not in title but certainly in duties.

Thanks to the novelty of a spring season and what seemed to be a pent-up demand for football following the NFL's strike-shortened 1982 season, the Express enjoyed a modicum of popularity in L.A. during the early stages of its first year despite a so-so start. We beat Herschel Walker and New Jersey 20-15 in our season opener but could manage nothing better than a 3-3 mark after six games. The USFL was a shaky proposition from Day One, but there is a certain glamour and glitz associated with being part of the L.A. sports scene, and the Express was no exception.

Our Hollywood connection was actor Lee Majors—the Six Million Dollar Man himself. An investor in the Express, Majors was no Jack Nicholson, but then we weren't exactly the Lakers. I assume part of Majors' interest in the Express stemmed from his own sports background. An all-state high school football player in Kentucky, Majors earned an athletic scholarship to Indiana before a back injury ended his playing career. Another thing about Majors: Contrary to what many believe, he is not related to former Tennessee and Pittsburgh football coach Johnny Majors.

Anyway, majority owners Alan Harmon and Bill Daniels held the Express' purse strings, but because of his celebrity status (such as it was) and football background, Majors served as a kind of figurehead owner that first year. Majors didn't associate with the coaches or players a whole lot, but I did have one opportunity to spend some time with him socially that spring following an Express victory.

After our 3-3 start we headed into a key Monday night matchup in Tampa Bay with the Central Division-leading Bandits and their offensive-minded coach Steve Spurrier, the 1966 Heisman Trophy winner from the University of Florida and the Gators' current head coach. Led by quarterback John Reaves and wide receiver Eric Truvillion, the 5-1 Bandits were one of the USFL's surprise teams in the early part of the season. As L.A.'s defensive coordinator, I knew we needed to keep the Bandit offensive unit off balance, so the other defensive coaches and I put together a series of blitzes and stunts designed to keep Reaves on his heels. Our plan worked extremely well; led by defensive back Mike Fox's three interceptions we held a 9-6 lead after three quarters. Then our defensive unit *really* came up big in the fourth quarter. On a Tampa Bay possession early in that final period, Reaves was forced out of the pocket and fumbled as he was hit near his own 20, suffering a broken wrist in the process. Defensive end Dennis Edwards recovered on the Bandits' 18-yard line, and four plays later running back John Bennett scored on a one-yard plunge to give us a 16-6 cushion. The Bandits cut our lead to 16-13 on a touchdown pass from backup quarterback Jimmy Jordan to Danny Buggs, but our defense scored a safety in the game's closing minutes and we pulled off a surprising 18-13 win. It was a stellar defensive effort and I received a fair amount of credit for L.A.'s victory that night.

A couple hours after the game I thought I'd have a quick celebratory beer before calling it a night, so I decided to check out the lounge at the hotel where the team was staying. As I walked in and bellied up to the bar, someone shouted, "Hey, Pokey!" I looked around but didn't see any familiar faces. Then I spotted Majors, who was sitting across the room, celebrating the Express' victory with a few companions. "Hey, Pokey!" he yelled again. "Great game! Let me buy you a drink!" I hesitated for half a second. "Uh ... sure, Lee," I finally said as I walked over to join Majors and his friends.

Pretty soon Majors was buying champagne for everyone at our table, and after an hour or two he and I were like lifelong friends. As our group dissected the game, toasted the Express' big win, and downed champagne I said to myself, "Hey, this pro football is great! Here I am partying with *Lee Majors!*" I really thought my career was going to take off and that I would be in the NFL in no time. Despite the rollicking good time I was having with Lee and the gang, I had to hit the sack because the coaching staff had to work the next day. Instead of returning to Los Angeles, the team was staying in Tampa for a couple more days, then traveling to Detroit later in the week to play Michigan on Saturday. With just four days between games, there was no rest for the coaches, and I had to get up early Tuesday to break down game films and devise a defensive package for the Panther offense.

The next morning I was walking by the hotel's pool, heading to a coaches' meeting when I heard a familiar voice yell, "Hey, Pokey!" At first I didn't see anyone, but then I looked up at a balcony on one of the hotel's penthouse suites. It was Majors. "Hey, Pokey!" he repeated. "Great time with ya last night! When we get back to California, I'll have you out to my place in Malibu and we'll have dinner or something!" I immediately had visions of Majors and his wife, Farrah Fawcett, and me and one of Farrah's girlfriends sitting in the Majors' hot tub, drinking champagne and having a great time. "Great, Lee!" I yelled back. "Give me a call after the Panthers game!" Me and Lee Majors, pals ... yeah, right. I should have known better.

Michigan wasn't exactly setting the world on fire going into our matchup in the Pontiac Silverdome. The Panthers dropped four of their first five games but had defeated Chicago 17-7 the day before our win in Tampa, improving their mark to 3-4. On film, the Michigan offense looked impressive in its win over the Blitz, but I still thought we were going to win. Unfortunately for us, the Panthers were in the early stages of a turn-around; they won 11 of their last 13 regular-season games and went on to claim the league championship. We led 17-13 at halftime, but the Panthers beat the tar out of us in the second half, winning 34-24. Both teams stood at 4-4.

Despite our identical marks, we were two teams going in opposite directions. While Michigan was on a roll, we struggled the remainder of the year. We never established any consistency and split our next six games, standing at 7-7 with four games remaining. The Pacific Division, however, was the weakest in the league. We were still in the hunt for the division title despite our lackluster performance. But the wheels fell off late in the season. We lost 42-17 in a rematch with Michigan, 20-13 to New Jersey, and 28-17 to lowly Washington, which entered our game with a league-worst 2-14 record. On the same day we lost to the Federals, Oakland clinched our division. We defeated Denver 21-14 on the final weekend to finish with an 8-10 mark, one game behind the Invaders, who qualified for the playoffs with a 9-9 record.

I never heard from Majors again.

The Invaders, whose defensive coordinator was Ron Lynn, my former colleague at Cal, lost to Michigan 37-21 in a first-round playoff game that drew more than 60,000 fans to the Silverdome. The Panthers beat Philadelphia 24-22 to claim the USFL's inaugural championship the following week. Part of the reason for the Panthers' title drive was their decision to ignore the USFL's salary cap as they raided the Pittsburgh Steelers' roster, signing guard Tyrone McGriff and tackle Ray Pinney. The USFL's strategy for player procurement emphasized, but did not mandate, a $1.3 million salary cap per team for the majority of the players each club signed, plus a more liberal policy to sign a "high-profile" player or two to enhance each team's—and the league's—credibility. But because the issue of a ceiling on player costs was never formally resolved, Michigan and some of the other free-spending franchises decided not to adhere to the $1.3 million guideline, much to the dismay of the more fiscally responsible owners, such as L.A.'s Harmon and Daniels.

HUGH CAMPBELL DIDN'T exactly turn heads his first year in L.A., but the recognition he garnered by coaching in the USFL seemed to enhance his credibility nonetheless; soon after the end of the NFL's 1983 season he was named head coach of the Houston Oilers. My premonition had come true. I figured I had finally gotten my big break.

But a day or so before Campbell was to announce who would be joining his staff in Houston, Keith Gilbertson got wind that he and I were the only Express assistants who were not going to be offered jobs; I didn't believe it. "Hey, Hugh's an intelligent guy," I said to Gilby. "It's not that the other guys can't coach, but we've got as much experience as most of them, and you and I know more about football than all those guys." I figured Gilby must have received some erroneous information. "Hugh wouldn't do something that stupid," I added.

But I was wrong, and he did. Campbell took every member of his staff to Houston with him except me and Gilbertson; to this day I'm not exactly sure why. Hugh could be a strange guy at times. I know it sounds like sour grapes when I say Gilby and I were the Express' best assistant coaches. But there was no question in my mind that we had as much if not more coaching ability than the people Campbell took to Houston. And between us, Gilby and I had almost 30 years' experience. (Keith began his coaching career in 1971 and had been the offensive coordinator for both Utah and Idaho before coming to the USFL.)

I was completely shocked. When I went into Campbell's office and asked him for an explanation, he just said he couldn't take me. That was it. I was so mad at the time, all I could say was, "I think you're making a mistake." In retrospect, it was just as well because Campbell compiled an 8-22 overall record in Houston and was fired by the Oilers before he completed his second year. He returned to Edmonton as the CFL team's general manager in 1986 and later interviewed me for the Eskimos' head coaching job following the 1990 season. I was a finalist for the job, and during my interview I again asked Campbell why he didn't take me and Gilbertson to Houston with him. He just laughed and said he had "other considerations," whatever the hell that meant.

To make matters worse, not only had Gilby and I been left behind, but we weren't retained by the Express—at least not initially—when the team was purchased in December of 1983 by San Francisco financier J. William Oldenburg. Oldenburg hired former Baltimore Colts and L.A. Rams general manager Don Klosterman as club president and GM. Klosterman, in turn, named John Hadl, a former AFL All-Star and NFL All-Pro quarterback with the San Diego Chargers and Los Angeles Rams, respectively, as the Express' head coach. Hadl, who had been the offensive coordinator for the University of Kansas, his alma mater, and quarterback coach for the Rams and the Denver Broncos before jumping to the USFL, knew little if anything about Gilbertson and me; we found out later that Campbell hadn't bothered to recommend either of us to Hadl before he left for the Oilers—another major source of irritation. Nevertheless, Gilby and I decided to offer our services to Hadl as he assumed the reins, providing information about players and hoping for a chance to be offered our old jobs back. One reason we stuck around was because most of Hadl's assistants were offensive coaches, including offensive coordinator and former Cal assistant Sam Gruneisen, and the team would eventually need some defensive assistants.

Hadl eventually hired Gilbertson to coach the defensive line; a few days later he told Gilby that he still needed a defensive coordinator and a defensive back coach. "Why don't you just hire Pokey?" Keith suggested. "He can do both." Good lord! I was only sitting under Hadl's nose. But I guess I should have been grateful when he offered me the job. With my rehiring by the Express, four refugees from Joe Kapp's Cal staff were co-ordinators in the USFL at the start of the 1984 season—me and Gruneisen in Los Angeles, Lynn in Oakland and Lary Kuharich, who was the offensive coordinator for the San Antonio Gunslingers. Another young coach trying to make a name for himself in the league was Al Borges, who served as a defensive assistant with the Invaders in 1984 and '85. Actually, Al was pulling double duty during that time. In the spring he worked with the Invaders, and in the fall he was the offensive coordinator for Diablo Valley College, a two-year school in Pleasant Hill, California.

In the next two seasons the USFL would continue to outbid the NFL and sign several more well-known college players, including the two Heisman Trophy winners to immediately follow Herschel Walker—Nebraska running back Mike Rozier with Pittsburgh in 1983 and Boston College quarterback Doug Flutie with New Jersey in '84. Other college standouts who began their careers in the USFL included quarterback Jim Kelly and running back Ricky Sanders of Houston, running back Gary Anderson and guard Nate Newton of Tampa Bay, Memphis defensive end Reggie White, New Orleans running back Marcus Dupree, and Jacksonville wide receiver Gary Clark.

As the 1984 season began, Oldenburg was determined to have a winning team in L.A. and spared no expense in signing the players he thought would help meet that objective. The Express signed two Nevada-Reno products, kicker Tony Zendejas and guard Derek Kennard, along with Purdue running back Mel Gray and Oregon offensive tackle Gary Zimmerman, all of whom became NFL standouts. Despite Oldenburg's willingness to spend vast amounts of money to sign top players, the Express was stuck in neutral as it started the 1984 season with two home losses—27-10 to Denver and 21-14 to Birmingham—in the Los Angeles

Coliseum. To make matters worse, fan interest seemed to be waning; after an encouraging turnout of 32,000 on opening day, the attendance at the Stallions game was less than 10,000. Despite the flagging interest in his team, Oldenburg made sports history the day after the Birmingham loss when he signed quarterback Steve Young for a staggering $40 million; at the time it was the highest contract ever paid to an athlete.

Six days later we played our first road game of the year, facing the defending division champ Invaders in the Oakland Coliseum. Both offenses were so inept that it looked like we would end in a scoreless tie. Young, who looked on in street clothes, must have wondered what he had gotten himself into as the Express offense turned the ball over six times in Oakland territory before Zendejas kicked a 40-yard field goal with four minutes remaining to give L.A. a 3-0 lead. With two minutes remaining we got the ball back near midfield; all quarterback Frank Seurer needed to do was take a knee a time or two to run out the clock and ensure the win. But for some reason Hadl instructed Seurer and the offense to try and score, which they did on a 13-yard run by Kevin Nelson with 1:07 remaining. "Gee, that was weird," I said to Gilbertson as we walked off the field after the 10-0 victory. "Why did we do that and risk a chance of losing the game? I don't understand." In the locker room afterward, Hadl awarded the game ball to our defense. While giving his postgame speech he praised just about every player and coach on the defensive unit except me—the damn defensive coordinator. I mean, I'm probably the last guy in the world to call attention to myself, but I thought this was pretty strange. I had just engineered what I thought was an outstanding game plan to help our team pitch a shutout and claim our first win of the season, yet it was like I was the invisible man in the locker room. "Gee," I muttered to myself during Hadl's speech, "this is weird."

During the entire return trip, Hadl never said a word to me. On the flight back to Los Angeles Klosterman and Hadl and their companions were seated in the first-class section of the plane while the players and assistants sat in coach; it sounded like they were having quite a party up front. While Klosterman and Hadl enjoyed the fruits of victory, I sat with Gilby and linebacker coach Mike Ackerley, eating some god-awful airline food and thinking how strange it was that no one else was invited to join the celebration.

We landed in L.A. and got on a bus, arriving at our team complex in Manhattan Beach around 10 p.m. Just as we were all getting ready to head to our homes, Hadl called me into his office. I walked in, thinking that he was finally going to say something positive, something like, "Hey, Pokey, great job. Hang in there. We all know your defense is playing great; we'll get the offense going and we'll make a run at it." Instead, he said, "Pokey, I hate to tell you this … but Klosterman told me to fire you."

I was floored. The only response I could come up with was, "You're shitting me? … I mean, didn't we just pitch a shutout?" But he didn't explain it any further. Dazed, I ran into Ackerley and Gilbertson outside Hadl's office. "Hey," I said, "Hadl just fired me." They looked at each other like I was joshing. But right away they could tell I wasn't. "You're shitting me?" Gilby said (that must have been the quote of the day). "What the hell for?"

I had no idea. I mean, out of 18 USFL teams, L.A.'s defense was ranked something like fifth statistically at the time. It just didn't make sense. Talk about star-crossed! I had some weird deals happen to me as a coach, but this one topped them all. I felt like the all-time leader on football's calamity list, a poster child for the vagaries of the coaching profession. In the early-morning hours of that same evening, I bought a bottle of wine and sat on the beach near the apartments where I lived and contemplated my future. I was pretty downcast, to say the least. It was time, I thought, to take inventory of my life and my career.

The next morning a secretary with the Express' front office came by my apartment to drop off the personal belongings I had left in my desk. "Here," she said, handing me a game ball from the previous night's contest. "The players wanted you to have this." The ball was signed by the Express players with an inscription that read something like, "Pokey Allen, defensive coordinator, L.A. 10, Oakland 0, March 11, 1984."

By the next day, the whole ugly affair began to make sense. Well, it still didn't make sense to me, but it sure illustrated the cruelties of the coaching business. Klosterman had ordered Hadl to fire me so that Ray Malavasi could have my job. Malavasi, head coach of the L.A. Rams from 1978-82, coached the Invaders' offensive line until Oakland head coach John Ralston dismissed him the week before the Express game. Six years earlier, Klosterman, then the Rams' GM, had hired Malavasi as the team's head coach; in 1982 Malavasi had hired Hadl as the Rams' quarterback coach. In other words, it was cronyism of the first order. I figure the old pals got together while the Express was in Oakland and decided good old Ray needed a job since he had just been fired by Ralston a few days earlier. I have no concrete proof, but in retrospect, I think I know why Hadl, who is now an associate athletic director at Kansas, ordered our offense to try and score that final touchdown against the Invaders: Firing a defensive coordinator after a 10-0 victory might raise a few less eyebrows than doing so after a 3-0 win. But, hey, that's life in the coaching business.

Hadl's explanation to the *Los Angeles Times* a couple of days later was as lame as the way the whole thing was handled. "It's not anything against Pokey," he told the paper. "He's done a good job. But with Ray sitting there, with the experience he's had, I felt like I had to do it. Pokey understood the best he could, I guess. It wasn't easy to do, believe me."

"It was a shock," I told the *Times*, "unbelievable, really. I'm sick about it." But since the Express was obligated to honor the remainder of my $60,000 contract, I thought it best not to complain too loudly. And so I began the longest period of unemployment in my life.

EVEN THOUGH I was drawing a paycheck from the Express, life without a job was really the pits. I'm not the type who can just sit around; after 17 seasons as a football coach, it was in my blood. The only period in my life that was more frustrating was the three months I spent in Vancouver in the fall of 1996 when I was undergoing alternative cancer treatment.

At night, I would stay up as late as I could so I would sleep in as late as I could the next morning. But I would invariably wake up at 7 a.m. anyway. Every morning I would work out and then walk over to a nearby Chinese restaurant to eat breakfast and to read the *L.A. Times*. I read everything, even the society pages; I could usually kill three hours reading the *Times*. Then I would go for a swim and work out some more. By then it was 5 or 6 p.m. Sometimes I'd start drinking around then, but if I started drinking too early, I'd go to bed by 9 or 10 and wake up at 3 in the morning. I mean, this unemployment was tough! It made for long days. After two months I started feeling like a grain of sand on a huge beach, which living in L.A. can do to you.

So I decided to pack up and move to my cabin at Flathead Lake. After all, I didn't have to pay rent there; besides, it was June by then and the weather was getting nicer in Montana. I borrowed Kim Williams' Volkswagen convertible (although we were no longer living together, we were still friends), loaded all of my worldly possessions into the car, drove down to the nearest bus depot, and put all my stuff on a bus to Missoula. A couple days later I took a plane to Missoula, picked up my stuff and hauled it to the cabin. You know, it's kind of sad when you're 41 years old and everything you own fits in a Volkswagen.

Even though I was on my own turf, I was still bored out of my mind. I briefly dabbled in real estate with my friend Ken Staninger but it wasn't to my liking; I think I was suffering from coaching withdrawal. I'll say one thing about being unemployed at that time: I was in the best shape of my life. In addition to training for another marathon I had purchased a bicycle and was logging some serious miles on it. On a typical day I would ride my bike the eight miles into Polson for breakfast. But unlike the *L.A. Times*, the Missoula newspaper was a quick read, 15 or 20 minutes at the most, which made for the start of a long day. One morning I was returning from breakfast, traveling downhill at a pretty good clip when I hit some loose gravel and wiped out less than a mile from the cabin. I went flying off the tree-lined road, smashing the bike and cutting my arm and my head. Dazed and bleeding, I had to carry the bike the rest of the way home because the collision bent the front wheel. "That's it," I said to myself. "I'm outta here."

Flathead Lake is a great place to live for a few weeks at a time, but I was going stir-crazy. I closed up the cabin, flew to Vancouver, and got an apartment the next day. I had several friends, including Jerry Bradley, still living in Vancouver. With my experience in the stock market, I was able to help Bradley a little with his stock promotion business, which he still does for a living. I stayed in Vancouver through the final six months of 1984 and into 1985. During that period I started going out with a woman from Vancouver named Diane Rees. We had first met when I was living in L.A but we didn't start dating until I was in Vancouver.

DURING MY HIATUS from coaching I should have taken a trip to Europe or some other faraway place. But my joblessness wouldn't allow such self-indulgence; if a coaching position was going to open up, I didn't want to miss the boat. After 17 years in the field I had plenty of connections and figured I'd land a job sooner or later, but I also knew how fickle the coaching business could be; the only person who was going to get me another job was me. In January 1985 I was still unemployed, so I decided to take my job search to the American Football Coaches Association's national conference in Nashville, Tennessee.

At those meetings I met up with Lary Kuharich, my former colleague at Cal who was now the Oakland Invaders' quarterback coach. Kuharich, who had been fired by San Antonio around the same time I got the ax from the Express, was from a football family which had connections that ran deep and wide. Lary's dad, the late Joe Kuharich, was a collegiate head coach at San Francisco and Notre Dame and an NFL head coach with the Chicago Cardinals, Washington Redskins and Philadelphia Eagles. At the time, Lary's brother Bill was the assistant general manager and director of player personnel for the USFL's Baltimore Stars. In 1986 Bill joined the New Orleans Saints' front office and today he is the NFL club's executive vice president and general manager.

Lary and I had become good friends since our days at Cal; in fact, he stayed with me for a while in Los Angeles between the time he got canned by the Gunslingers and hired by the Invaders. "We were just a couple of coaches looking for work," Kuharich told a reporter years later when asked to recall the time we roomed together after we both lost our jobs in 1984. "We were both feeling pretty low at the time, but I think we picked up each other's spirits. And Pokey was good at that. I'll tell you what, it was hard being dejected around him. Pokey was a real friend." (Lary later served as head coach for the CFL's Calgary Stampeders and the B.C. Lions; the past several years he has coached in the Arena Football League and the World League of American Football. In four seasons he guided the Tampa Bay Storm to a 31-23 record and won the ArenaBowl championship in 1993. In 1996 he was named head coach of the league's New York CityHawks.)

As luck would have it, Lary knew Dick Coury, the head coach of the USFL's Portland Breakers who was also at the coaches' meetings in Nashville. It just so happened that the Breakers, who were moving to their third city in as many years, were in need of a defensive coordinator. As Kuharich introduced us, Coury shook my hand and politely listened to my pitch, but he didn't seem the least bit interested in me. Coury was a veteran coach with a solid reputation; the same couldn't be said, however, for his team. In a league rife with instability, the Breakers were the most nomadic of all USFL franchises. In 1983 Coury had earned USFL Coach of the Year honors for guiding the overachieving Boston Breakers to a respectable 11-7 record and having them in the playoff hunt until the closing weeks of the season. But because fan interest in Boston was tepid, owner Joe Canizaro, a real estate and commercial properties developer, moved the franchise to New Orleans for the '84 season.

The change of scenery, however, failed to improve the team's sorry situation. With the exception of first-year running back Marcus Dupree, an underclassman out of the University of Oklahoma whom many considered the second coming of Herschel Walker, the Breakers continued to be a team of marginal talent. Nevertheless, Coury's magic from the previous year continued into the first half of the '84 season as New Orleans won its first five games and surged to a 7-2 record at the halfway point, good for second place in the Eastern Conference's Southern Division. But the club would win just one game the entire second half, finishing 8-10. Not only did the Breakers fizzle on the field, but their financial situation did not improve in New Orleans. As was the case in Boston, the Breakers had trouble putting fans in the seats; only this time the venue was the high-rent Superdome. The lack of fan support and the team's inability to compete with the NFL's Saints proved to be too big a task; in November of 1984 Canizaro announced that he was moving his team to Portland, Oregon. Although I was willing to take a job almost anywhere, my interest in the Breakers was heightened by the fact they would be in the Pacific Northwest.

After we met in Nashville, I called Coury a time or two to inquire about the vacancy on his staff; his reaction was lukewarm at best. "No," he told me, he hadn't made his selection yet. "Of course," he replied, he would keep me in mind. "Yes," he wearily intoned, he had my phone number in Vancouver. I was getting the distinct impression that I was not at the top of Coury's list. With the start of the USFL's 1985 preseason training camps rapidly approaching, I was starting to become even more concerned because the few assistant coaching positions that were still open were quickly being filled. I thought I had a shot at the defensive coordinator's position with the Denver Gold, but head coach Mouse Davis selected Joe Haering instead.

Given Coury's apparent indifference toward me, I was pretty surprised when he called me in late January, just a week or so before the opening of the Breakers' training camp in Pomona, California. "Pokey," he said, "are you still looking for work?" I flew down to Los Angeles and eagerly signed on as Portland's defensive coordinator about five days before the start of preseason drills. Coaching and management changes were a common occurrence in the uncertain and unstable world of the USFL, especially between the 1984 and '85 seasons. And with each transaction you could often find an ironic twist; my new job with Portland certainly had one: Breakers president John Ralston.

Among the many changes in the USFL in 1985 was the merger of the Oakland and Michigan franchises; with the Michigan faction assuming the principal ownership, Ralston, the Invaders' coach, was the odd man out. But he soon found work as Portland's chief executive. I first crossed paths with Ralston following my senior season of high school football in the fall of 1960 when he unsuccessfully tried to recruit me to play for him at Utah State. Now, nearly a quarter of a century later, I was finally in his employ. Furthermore, it was Ralston's dismissal of Ray Malavasi the previous season in Oakland that precipitated my ouster in Los Angeles.

Anyway, I was delighted to be joining the Breakers, but my late arrival immediately put our defense in a bind. We had a preseason game scheduled February 9 against Denver followed by another exhibition against L.A. a week later, and I simply didn't have an adequate amount of time to assess our personnel and prepare a decent playbook. I hastily threw together a game plan for our contest against the Gold, but Davis' run-and-shoot offense was too much for our ill-prepared defense as Denver quarterback Vince Evans threw a pair of touchdown passes to lead his team to a 27-9 win. Our defensive unit fared even worse the following week against Los Angeles as Steve Young threw for a touchdown and ran for another in a 38-17 Express win.

After our two exhibition losses I was able to pinpoint part of our defense unit's problem: We were just plain bad. Even so, it was ultimately my responsibility as defensive coordinator to get results, which caused me to wonder whether I was going to get fired before the regular season even started. I think I might have been paranoid after what happened to me the previous year in L.A. Man, I was sweating after those two preseason blowouts. But that didn't stop me from doing everything I could to turn things around. Our coaching staff put in incredibly long hours—sometimes going from 6:30 in the morning till well past midnight—in preparation for our regular-season opener in Arizona.

In spite of our shortcomings in the talent department, our defensive coaches were finally able to fully assess our personnel and install a solid defensive plan for the Outlaw offense and quarterback Doug Williams. Going into our game in Sun Devil Stadium, I anticipated a much-improved performance by our defense, and I was right. Williams completed 16 of 26 passes for 254 yards, but we managed to hold Arizona without a touchdown. Unfortunately, we still lost 9-7 as Outlaw kicker Luis Zendejas booted three field goals. After such a great defensive effort we were terribly disappointed, but our problems were only beginning: Marcus Dupree blew out his knee in the second quarter and was lost for the season.

Our next contest was the Breakers' Portland debut on March 2 against the L.A. Express, which lost its season opener 34-33 to Jim Kelly and the Houston Gamblers. Our Monday night home opener would mark the first pro football game in Portland since the WFL's Thunder played there a decade earlier, and the whole city was fired up. But our club had some big problems; not only had we lost our franchise player, but many of the players had no place to stay when we arrived in Portland following the Arizona game. Because the Breakers had moved from New Orleans, held their training camp in the L.A. area and played their season opener in Tempe, about 90 percent of the players had never set foot in Portland prior to our arrival. We were totally disorganized. Instead of preparing for the Express, many of the players spent those first few days in Portland looking for apartments and unpacking. Coury was one of the few members of the team who was familiar with Portland; in 1974 he was the head coach of the WFL's Portland Storm, which was reorganized and renamed the Thunder the following year. I initially stayed with linebacker coach Bob Shaw until I found a place to live. Later I roomed with Breakers marketing executive Steve "Dream" Weaver, one of the few holdovers from the Breakers' front office when they were in New Orleans.

To compound our concerns, we figured the Express, considered one of the top teams in the USFL at the start of the season, would be loaded for bear following its tough opening-day loss. And given the way Young and Company had clobbered us in our exhibition contest a few weeks earlier, we knew we needed to make some major adjustments if we were to have any chance of winning—especially with Dupree on the sidelines. Express coach John Hadl seemed to think as much. "We should win it, no question about it," he told the *Los Angeles Times* when asked about his club's upcoming game in Portland.

But I thought we could beat the Express. Having been L.A.'s defensive coordinator for all of 1983 and part of the previous season, I had a pretty good idea how to exploit what few weaknesses the Express offense had. Moreover, based on Young's performance in our preseason matchup, I designed several other adjustments that I thought might work to offset his strengths. Young's arm with the Express in 1985 had not developed to what it is with the San Francisco 49ers today. In addition, it was only his second year in pro ball so he was still pretty inexperienced. What we did that Monday evening in Portland was rush three and drop eight players back into pass coverage. We would occasionally rush four players at Young, but for the most part he was forced to throw into a secondary swarming with linebackers and defensive backs. I don't think he had ever faced a defense like the one we threw at him that night.

In front of a raucous Civic Stadium crowd of more than 25,000 fans, our defense forced three fumbles and an interception and made Young's life miserable the entire game en route to a surprising 14-10 win. Young ran for more than 100 yards that night, scoring L.A.'s lone touchdown when he ducked two tackles on a nine-player blitz and ran it in from eight yards out. Steve Young is one of the best running quarterbacks I have ever seen—a tremendous scrambler. I couldn't believe how damn fast he was back then.

But we stymied the rest of the Express offense, and in our first two games our defense had given up just one TD. In the coaching business you learn not to take things too personally, but given the way I was treated

by the Express the previous season, I'd have to say that victory was especially satisfying. Still, it's never been my nature to gloat. "Beating L.A. was
a great win for us—in more ways than one," was the only comment I made
when a reporter asked me if I had derived any special pleasure in our win
over the Express. After the game team owner Joe Canizaro was so pleased
and excited that he loaned the coaching staff his private limousine so we
could go out and celebrate. So there I was, driving through downtown
Portland in the owner's limo, thinking once again that I was pretty hot
stuff, how I had orchestrated two nearly flawless defensive packages, how
I was about to forge my reputation as a defensive whiz, and how it was
only a matter of time before some NFL team would snap me up.

But like the other times, my illusion of grandeur was short-lived; our
upset win over L.A. that night turned out to be one of the rare highlights
in a season full of financial problems and inept performances. Without
Dupree, our running game was the pits. We split our first four games and
then fell to 2-3 with a 27-20 loss in Houston. I thought our defense played
pretty well against Jim Kelly in that contest, even though he threw a pair
of touchdown passes. After the seventh week we stood at 3-4 following a
30-17 win over Oakland.

Moreover, money woes were running rampant through the USFL. I
didn't realize how bad things had gotten until we met the Express in the
L.A. Coliseum in late April. Beset by fiscal problems after Bill Oldenburg
relinquished his ownership after some questionable financial dealings, the
Express was a team in turmoil with scant financial backing and dwindling
fan support. The Express defeated us 17-12, but what I remember most
about that game is how empty the Coliseum seemed. I don't recall what
the attendance was that day, but I'll bet there weren't more than a couple
thousand people there. It was just awful, an embarrassment.

And things got worse for our club. The following week we suffered
a 45-7 home-field loss to Houston as Kelly threw for 348 yards and four
touchdowns. Two weeks later we dropped a 30-21 decision to Arizona in
front of 15,275, the smallest crowd of the year in Portland's Civic Stadium.
The following week we ended a six-game losing streak with a 17-14 win
over Memphis on the strength of six interceptions, the last of which set up
Tim Mazzetti's game-winning 44-yard field goal as time expired.

The Breakers were no exception to the fiscal problems that plagued
the USFL in 1985. More than once, paychecks were delayed, and with about
four weeks remaining in the season management told the coaching staff
that we probably weren't going to get paid the rest of the year. To make
matters worse, the assistant coaches were told to break the news to the

players. We tried to sell them on the belief that if they ever wanted to play pro ball anywhere else, they better hang in there—even though we knew it was a bunch of bullshit. The players stayed on, but our morale was low, to say the least. We somehow managed to win two of our final four games, but by June 1985 the future of the entire USFL was in serious doubt. We went winless on the road that year and finished fifth in the USFL's seven-team Western Conference with a 6-12 record; it was small consolation that the Express finished behind us with a 5-13 mark.

Once again I found myself in a strange situation when Canizaro informed the players and coaches that he couldn't pay us. I basically had a year and a half remaining on a personal services contract that called for an annual salary of $60,000, which meant the Breakers owed me about $90,000. Canizaro was trying to reach a settlement with his coaches with one lump sum, but I was getting pretty tired of all the crap and wanted to fight for the full amount. Some of my fellow assistant coaches, however, were in bad shape financially and had families and other concerns, so I agreed to go along with their wishes; we reached a settlement with Canizaro and I got about $9,000 of the $90,000 he owed me. I wasn't the only one who got fleeced by Canizaro; he owed a ton of money to a long list of creditors who did business with the Breakers during their lone year in Portland.

At the conclusion of the 1985 season I spent several weeks in Vancouver to be with Diane Rees and visit Bradley and other friends. But for the most part I stayed in Portland and lived in a rented house with Dream Weaver because I was told the USFL would be making a last-gasp effort to stay alive.

With the Breakers' financial demise and the future of the USFL in question, I was once again unemployed and living a life that was considerably less than extravagant. When I was with the Breakers I had a complimentary car, but now all Weaver and I had was a second-hand Chrysler that I think he finagled from a local dealer. We were so financially strapped we didn't even have a garbage can and dumped our rubbish in a trash bin behind a nearby building. Weaver was also unemployed at the time, but at least he owned a TV and some other furniture. Despite our situation we managed to laugh a lot. Quite often our Sunday entertainment was nothing more than buying some beer and settling in front of the television for the worst movie we could find. We watched some of the all-time bad sci-fi films on TV during those months. When the USFL eventually folded, Weaver and I went into the Breakers' office and, um ... relieved the team of some stuff it no longer needed, including a projector and the Breakers sign on the office wall.

With the USFL's demise I once again sought work in the NFL, but the competition, as always, was tough. I had a few contacts, including San Francisco defensive coordinator George Seifert and Philadelphia assistant Lynn Stiles, both former teammates of mine at Utah who I hoped could help me out. Both Seifert, who later became the 49ers' head coach, and Stiles, now a vice president with the Kansas City Chiefs, said they would keep their eyes open, but nothing ever panned out.

Then in December of 1985 Coury called me and suggested I apply for the head coaching job at Portland State, which had opened up when Don Read took the head job at the University of Montana. Coury said he knew then-PSU president Joseph Blumel and would recommend me for the position if I was interested. I wasn't really excited about re-entering the college ranks at the time, but my efforts to find work in the NFL had been fruitless up to that point, so figured I would give it a shot. I took Coury's advice, got my résumé together and applied.

For once, something good was about to happen.

Chapter 9

A Program in Portland

Portland State University. In 1986 it wasn't exactly synonymous with college football excellence. The Vikings had forged a reputation as a small-college offensive juggernaut under head coach Mouse Davis from 1975-80 with future NFL quarterbacks June Jones (1975-76) and Neil Lomax (1977-80) at the controls. But the PSU football program had fallen on hard times under Don Read, who replaced Davis in 1981. When Read left for Montana at the conclusion of the '85 season, the fifth year of his second stint at the Vikings' helm, he had just one winning season and a 19-33-1 overall record. (Read was 20-19 in his first go-round as PSU's head coach from 1968-71.)

Like most Division II football programs, PSU operated on a small amount of capital; to make matters worse, attendance figures were on the decline. From 1975-80 Davis' high-scoring teams drew an average of 5,924 fans to Portland's Civic Stadium, but the average attendance fell to 3,863 during Read's second tour of duty. Furthermore, Joseph Blumel, a supporter of the football program throughout his presidency at Portland State, was preparing to retire, adding further doubt to the program's stability.

Terry Frei, then a columnist with the *Oregonian*, Portland's daily newspaper, later wrote that there were "mixed, even depressing signals about [the future of] football from the soon-to-be-gone PSU administration" when the school began its search for Read's replacement. If one word could sum up the general sentiments toward the PSU football program at the time, it would be apathy. "PSU football was decent for its level, but moribund," Frei wrote. "On the interest scale, it was nowhere." Frei, who now writes for the *Denver Post*, added that Read was "a good coach who had tired of fighting the Division II battles on a shoestring and understandably wondered whether the program could survive."

Like I said, my initial reaction to Dick Coury's recommendation that I apply for the PSU position was one of ambivalence. But the more I thought about it, the more the job appealed to me. Besides, it wasn't like NFL teams were beating a path to my door to vie for my services. My co-head coaching experience at Simon Fraser notwithstanding, I had never been a *real* head coach before, and I *was* interested in trying something new. Besides, I *really* needed a job because Steve Weaver had decided to start a marketing and promotions business in his hometown of St. Louis and was getting ready to move out of the house we shared, which would leave me with all the rent payments.

Thanks to Coury I got my foot in the door, but as I was going through the interview process I got the distinct impression I wasn't the selection committee's top choice; that distinction went to Western Oregon State head coach Duke Iverson. Sure enough, after interviewing the candidates the committee recommended Iverson for the job. But it was Blumel's call, and the PSU president did a curious thing: He politely rejected the committee's choice and picked me. I guess he was a good judge of character. Around the second week of January Blumel called and offered me the job while I was in the Bay Area at the 1986 East-West Shrine Game, still trying to hook up with George Seifert and Lynn Stiles to see if they knew of any NFL job openings. I had some concerns about the program's stability and really didn't look at the position as all that great a career move. But I wasn't in a position to be picky so I accepted the offer. Just a few months after I was hired, Blumel retired as PSU president and athletic director Roy Love stepped down to return to teaching at the university.

I started at an annual salary of about $40,000. In contrast to the media circus that would take place seven years later in Boise when I was named head coach at Boise State, the announcement that I was PSU's new football coach barely caused a ripple in Portland. With the NBA's headline-grabbing Trail Blazers and Pac-10 schools Oregon and Oregon State to contend with, Viking football wasn't a real high priority with Portland's press back then.

But with the program in such sorry shape at the time, I was almost thankful for the limited media attention. I mean, despite my public remarks to the contrary when I got hired, I wasn't exactly brimming with optimism when I took the job. Like I said, PSU football had not done well, either at the gate or in the Western Football Conference standings in the mid-80s; the Vikings went 4-5-1 under Read the previous fall and averaged a little more than 4,000 fans per game. To make matters worse, I had only 20 scholarships and a limited budget to work with. Plus, the prime recruiting weeks had already passed and I still had to select my assistant coaches.

I started by hiring two holdovers from Read's staff—offensive line coach Dave Stromswold and defensive back coach Rick Olson, a part-timer the previous two seasons. My next step was to select my two coordinators. Both of my first choices declined my offer, so I ended up hiring fellow USFL refugee Al Borges to guide the offense and Eastern Washington linebacker coach Tom Mason to direct the defense. Borges was a fellow assistant coach during my one year at Cal who went on to work with the USFL's Oakland Invaders in 1984 and '85 while Mason and I coached together at EWU in 1981. As it turned out, I'm glad my first choices turned me down because I wound up with two of the finest coordinators in college football—and two close friends with whom I would share some of the greatest moments of my career. I rounded out the staff by hiring three more coaches—Washington State graduate assistant Tom Osborne for the running backs, Lewis and Clark College assistant Bill Hartman for the special teams, and Barry Sacks for the defensive line. Sacks, who was coaching in Washington's high school ranks at the time, was one of my favorite players when I was an assistant at Montana; I figured he would bring the same intensity to our program that he brought to the field as a player—and I was right.

My new assistants certainly didn't join PSU's program for the money. Borges' and Mason's starting salaries were $20,500 while Sacks, Osborne and Olson started at a measly $8,000 apiece. Luckily, the income wasn't all that important because all of us were single except for Mason, whose wife, Jami Reilly, had a teaching job in Spokane. (She joined Tom in Portland when the school year ended.) Given everyone's shaky financial situation, it was decided that Borges, Mason and Sacks would join Weaver and me in the three-bedroom house we were renting on 65th Street in Portland, about six miles from the PSU campus. A few weeks later Weaver left for St. Louis, which gave us a little more room. Actually, it gave us a *lot* more room because Steve took all his furniture with him.

Once again, I found myself in what I thought was a pretty amusing—some might call it pitiful—situation. I mean, all I could do was laugh. Here I was, a 43-year-old refugee from a defunct football league, trying to revive a languishing college program with a limited budget, having no transportation (Weaver took his car too), and living in a house that had no furniture with three guys in worse financial shape than me. Seriously now, how much goofier could it get? But you know what? We had a great time despite our meager accommodations. We were on the road recruiting, getting ready for spring drills, and just having a great time trying to get the football program rolling. It was hard work that required long hours and we took our jobs seriously, but we also made the time to laugh and have fun—big time. I could recount some pretty wild and earthy stories that took place during those three or four months we lived together, but I think some tales are better left untold. Suffice it to say, we weren't a delicate or prudish bunch.

I already had one of the bedrooms, but the sleeping arrangements weren't so great for the others. Borges laid claim to Weaver's bedroom, but Al had to sleep on the living room couch until Dream moved out. Mason and Sacks didn't have beds and had to use sleeping bags, but at least Tom had a bedroom. With the sofa now gone (Weaver didn't leave us a damn thing), Sacks was relegated to what served as the remaining sleeping quarters—the laundry room. Mason eventually grew weary of sleeping on the floor and bought two 99-cent blow-up air mattresses for himself and Sacks to put under the sleeping bags. The rest of our furniture consisted of a couple of metal folding chairs and a few cheap plastic chairs that we "borrowed" from the PSU football offices.

By this time I had been dating Diane Rees for about a year. She worked in the travel industry, so it was relatively easy and inexpensive for her to fly down from Vancouver, which she did most weekends. However, our long-distance relationship was becoming a real aggravation, so in the spring she moved from Vancouver to be with me in Portland. Problem was, our decision to cohabit was a package deal with the three other guys. We all knew the whole situation in the house was temporary, but after a few weeks of living in a small house with four men—none of whom you would call quiet or bashful—it came as no surprise when Diane told me she was having trouble adjusting to her new digs. Later that spring we all decided it was time for our happy little family to split up. Mason's wife finished the school year and joined him in Portland, Sacks and Borges got an apartment, and Diane and I moved onto a houseboat on the Columbia River.

I bought the houseboat because I thought it would be a good investment and a fun place to live; besides I've always been a little unconventional. Located near Portland's Jantzen Beach with about 250 other houseboats, our new home had all the comforts of a typical house without the hassles of lawn care or other domestic chores that I've never enjoyed. The only problem was the houseboat needed some interior work. Lucky for me Mason is a pretty talented carpenter and was willing to remodel the place for me. He gutted the inside and took the old boatwell—a garagelike slip that was attached to the main structure—and converted it into a living room, kitchen and utility room. He also replaced the boatwell's garage door with a picture window that looked out onto the river. It was easily a $15,000 job that Tom did for $1,000.

It was a great place to live, a lot like the houseboat in the movie *Sleepless in Seattle*. It was about 1,400 square feet with a 900-square-foot deck that was perfect for large barbecues and parties. Having that houseboat made a huge difference with our fund-raising efforts because it was a great place to entertain boosters and other people.

The houseboat, however, was not really a place conducive to my somnambulation. As I mentioned before, I've been known to sleepwalk. As a kid, I would occasionally wander the house at night—sound asleep. Back then it wasn't a problem; my mom would hear me, get up and steer me back to bed. But as an adult living on a boat, it was a little more hazardous. About 10 times a year—more so, it seems, during football season when the tension is high—I take nocturnal strolls. One night after Jerry Bradley and I had a party on the houseboat, I went to bed with my jeans on. The next morning I woke up to find the jeans soaking wet on the living room floor. I couldn't understand how they got there and why they were wet. Bradley and a couple of friends who had spent the night told me that I had gotten up in the middle of the night, walked onto the deck and stepped right off—straight into the drink. Amid howls of laughter, they said I then pulled myself out of the water, wandered back into the living room, took off my sopping-wet pants, and returned to bed without waking up. "Bullshit," I said. "How can a guy sleepwalk into the water and get up and come back to bed without remembering it?" Bradley was laughing so hard he could hardly reply. "How the hell should I know," he said. "You're the one who did it."

OK, I admit it, I *do* sleepwalk. The first thing I do when I go to bed in a hotel now is lock myself in. Because if I get up to go to the bathroom and I'm not fully awake … well, let's just say I don't want to have a repeat performance of what happened in Everett, Washington. I've been told I've tried to open a sliding glass door in a hotel room in my sleep. Actually, I'm surprised I haven't tried to walk off a balcony! It's scary.

Anyway, after living together on the houseboat for about a year and a half, Diane and I got engaged in the fall of 1987. But neither of us could take the plunge; at issue were our conflicting views on what we wanted out of marriage. Fourteen years my junior, Diane wanted kids. But I was nearly 45 and not particularly interested in raising a family in my middle-aged years (an attitude I decidedly changed when my daughter was born five years later). Another potential problem was Diane's belief that I would probably devote more time and effort to my career than to our marriage—a concern that was not totally unjustified. We broke up in February 1988, and she eventually moved back to Vancouver. Like most of my ex-girl-friends, Diane, whose last name is now Hemingson, and I remained friends and keep in touch. She now lives in Whistler, British Columbia, with her husband and two kids.

TO SAY I got off to an inauspicious start as a head coach in the fall of 1986 would be an understatement. In my PSU debut we lost to the University of Idaho in Moscow 42-10. Interestingly, my opposite number that day was my friend Keith Gilbertson, who was also making his head coaching debut. Gilby had been an assistant under Dennis Erickson and took over the UI program when Erickson left after the 1985 season for the head job at the University of Wyoming. Our second contest, a 51-14 loss to UNLV in Las Vegas, was equally one-sided. Having been outscored 93-24 in our first two games, it initially looked like 1986 was going to be a long season. But then we got our act together and reeled off three straight home wins—27-21 over Weber State, 27-16 over Humboldt State and 41-17 over Southern Utah in our Western Football Conference opener. A 52-20 whipping by eventual league champ Sacramento State evened our WFC mark at 1-1 and our overall record at 3-3 after six weeks.

We then went on another three-game winning streak—beating Cal Lutheran 28-7, Cal Poly-San Luis Obispo 66-7 and Santa Clara 41-14—before dropping our final two contests—34-0 to Cal State-Northridge and 35-14 to Don Read and Montana.

All in all, I'd say my first year as a head coach wasn't a total disaster. Our overall record was an unimpressive 6-5, but we did end up grabbing a share of second place in the WFC with a 4-2 league mark. Our average attendance that year, 4,891, improved by nearly 900 per game from the previous season, a small increase but an increase nonetheless. We didn't exactly blow our opponents off the field, but our offense played an entertaining brand of football and three key performers from that squad—center Dave Swanson, quarterback Chris Crawford and tight end Barry Naone—were among our returning players for 1987. Crawford finished his sophomore year ranked seventh nationally in passing efficiency among Division II quarterbacks while Naone, also a sophomore, was second in the nation with 62 receptions. In addition, running back Kevin Johnson set a single-season school rushing record with 902 yards.

It was a good thing we finished above .500 our first year because I don't think new PSU president Natale Sicuro, who replaced the retired Blumel in September of 1986, was all that impressed with me or our football team. Sicuro was a strong-willed administrator who I think would have preferred to bring in his own coach. But since we had a "winning" season our first year, I think he had to take a wait-and-see attitude. (I would compare Sicuro's forceful management style to that of John Keiser, Boise State's former president. But at least Keiser had a personality.) By the end of the following season, however, the football staff's job security was not an issue because we won—big time.

Some of the similarities between our second season at Portland State in 1987 and our second year at Boise State in '94 were not a coincidence. In both cases our staff endured a rocky first season after which we assessed our strengths and weaknesses and identified our needs. In both cases we brought in junior college transfers to shore up our biggest deficiencies. And in both cases we were dynamite.

NO QUESTION ABOUT it, 1987 was a watershed year in my coaching career. But what transpired on the football field that autumn and early winter was only part of the story. That's because 1987 also marked the beginning of my starring role in a series of imaginative publicity stunts designed to sell PSU football tickets. I didn't realize it at the time, but those TV commercials and related promotions would help shape my public persona. Steve Weaver, who returned to Portland in 1988 as PSU's director of marketing and promotions, came up with plenty of wacky ideas in an effort to market our football program. But the person who started our off-the-wall TV spots in 1987 was PSU booster Cap Hedges, owner of a Portland advertising agency. Hedges, a Portland State alumnus, had volunteered his talent and resources to write and produce the yearly TV commercials for Viking football ticket sales since the mid-70s. In 1986 he did some promotional videos using me, some crowd shots and "The Hokeypokey" song, but I thought the whole thing was just *too* hokey.

Then in the spring of 1987 Cap decided it might be a good idea to try and sell PSU football tickets by using my—um, what's the right word here?—unique personality. He wrote three scripts for my review. The first was pretty straightforward, the second was a little offbeat, and the third was pretty goofy. I chose the third—and a star was born.

The commercial showed a bunch of Viking players running and tackling, and in the corner of the picture my face appeared; I pointed at the camera and yelled: "I'm Portland State Viking football coach Pokey Allen! If you don't buy your season tickets now, a big meteor will land in your backyard!" I can't remember if those were the exact words, but it was something like that. The funny thing was it caught on; all of a sudden we started selling a few more season tickets. Not a lot at the outset, but sales were improving.

"Pokey had a knack for those spots; he just seemed to have a twinkle in his eye when he did them," Hedges told a writer a few years later. "That one spot in 1987 really kicked off his image—and promoted the program at the same time. Each spring we would do a new spot, and in the springs to follow, we would have Pokey do things like ride an elephant, get shot from a cannon, and walk through a wall of fire. Our commercials became media events in themselves. We had TV crews filming us filming Pokey."

More important, we started winning that fall. Led by Crawford on offense and linemen Brent Napierkowski and Anthony Spears, two of our 21 JC imports, on defense, we thought we had the potential to have an outstanding team in 1987. We opened the season at home with a 33-7 win over Wisconsin-Stevens Point; the attendance, however, was a disappointing 3,648. I think the people in Portland sat up and took notice the following week when we traveled to Montana and ambushed the Grizzlies 20-3. But in that game we lost Kevin Johnson to a knee injury. The next week was a home game against Keith Gilbertson and Idaho, which we lost 17-10 before 8,535 fans, the second-largest PSU football crowd in Civic Stadium since 1980.

Then we started to roll. We routed Southern Utah 38-6 and Humboldt State 50-14 before playing to a 24-24 tie with Idaho State in Pocatello. Mason's defensive unit had played extremely well through our first six games, but in our next four contests it was indomitable. We blanked Sac State 40-0, limiting the Hornets to 179 yards total offense and avenging our lopsided loss in Sacramento the previous year. We then beat Cal Lutheran 40-7, Cal Poly-SLO 31-7 and Santa Clara 41-0.

Despite our 8-1-1 record, our football program still hadn't entirely caught on in Portland. Our average attendance was only 5,000 per game going into our regular-season finale with Cal State-Northridge. And in spite of what we had accomplished to that point, a loss to the Matadors would all but ruin our season. Our league record was 5-0 while Northridge was 3-1; if the Matadors could beat us and defeat Sacramento State the following week, they would earn a share of the league championship. Furthermore, a loss to Northridge would severely hurt, if not kill, our chances of getting one of the eight invitations to the NCAA Division II playoffs.

That's when I decided to contact Norm Daniels, president of G.I. Joe's, a Portland-based sporting goods and automotive retail chain. Hedges had earlier introduced Daniels to me and PSU football, and I got to know Norm and several other business types while socializing with them at Jake's, a popular Portland restaurant. During that time Daniels had become a solid backer of our program. "Norm," I begged, "you've got to help us out." I asked Daniels if he would take out a full-page ad in the *Oregonian* and basically tell the people of Portland that they had to help us get to the playoffs because if we could beat Northridge *and* draw a big crowd, there was a chance we could actually host a first-round game. Not only did Daniels agree to buy the ad, his store gave out G.I. Joe "touchdown" towels for fans to wave at the game.

On November 14 we finally had a game with a playoff atmosphere: a large crowd (nearly 12,000), a formidable opponent (Northridge was a respectable 6-3 overall and had routed us the previous year), and a league championship and possible playoff berth on the line. On our first possession, running back Curtis Delgardo, a 5-foot-5 sophomore who replaced the injured Johnson after the second game of the year, raced 69 yards for a touchdown, giving us a quick 7-0 lead. Northridge fought back, however, and our lead was a precarious 24-16 going into the final quarter. Spurred by the big crowd, we scored two fourth-quarter touchdowns and pulled away for a 38-22 victory. Crawford threw for 235 yards and two TDs, both to wide receiver Tim Corrigan, and Delgardo finished with 124 yards on the ground. We captured the WFC title with a 6-0 record and finished the regular season at 9-1-1. Without Daniels and G.I. Joe's, I'm not sure we could have pulled it off. In my opinion, Norm Daniels helped save Portland State football that day.

After six years of mostly listless football, Portland State came out of nowhere in 1987. But we were no fluke. At the conclusion of the regular season Mason's defense was ranked second in the nation among Division II schools, yielding just 9.7 points per game, while Borges' offensive unit averaged 31.7 points a game, good for fifth place nationally. Crawford, who finished fourth in the balloting for the nation's Division II Player of the Year award, completed 191 of 294 passes for a school-record 65 percent while Delgardo also established a PSU mark with 1,046 yards rushing. Crawford and free safety Tracey Eaton were the WFC's Offensive and Defensive Player of the Year, respectively.

As we awaited an invitation to the Division II playoffs, I thought our chances of hosting a first-round game were pretty good because our average attendance ended up being slightly more than 6,100, not bad by Division II standards. I can remember the promoter in me thinking, "Please, God, give us an opponent with a state in its name—Northern Colorado,

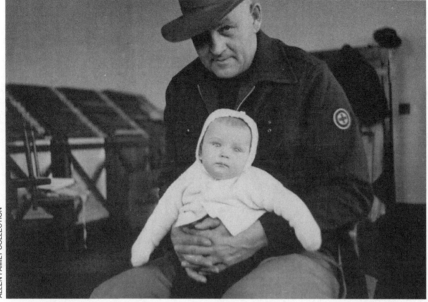

ALLEN FAMILY COLLECTION

Pokey Allen Jr. and Sr., late 1943. Pokey Sr. was a 23-year veteran of the Montana Highway Patrol.

With sister Jennie and family pet Oscar, circa 1946.

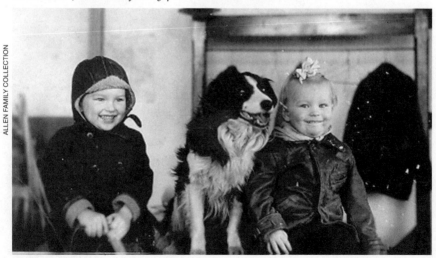

ALLEN FAMILY COLLECTION

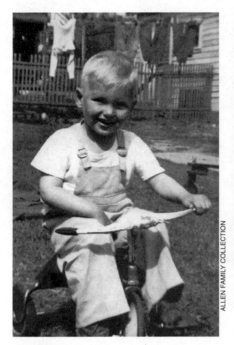

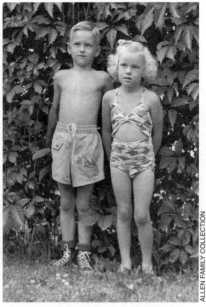

A toddler growing up in Missoula.

Making a summer fashion statement with Jennie in the late 1940s. Big brother and little sister were only 18 months apart in age.

With Mom, Jennie and Dad, flashing the form that would later bring gridiron glory.

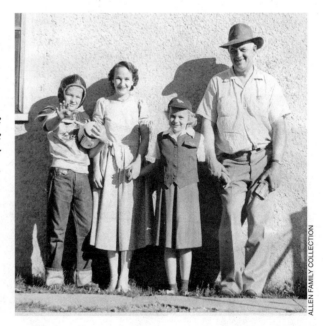

Here's the 14-year-old slugger playing for the KXLL Knights of the Missoula Babe Ruth League.

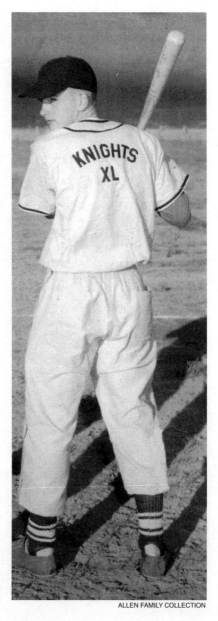

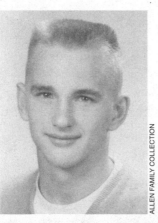

ALLEN FAMILY COLLECTION

The clean-cut, All-American kid in junior high.

ALLEN FAMILY COLLECTION

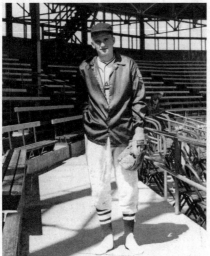

ALLEN FAMILY COLLECTION

A member of Missoula's American Legion baseball team.

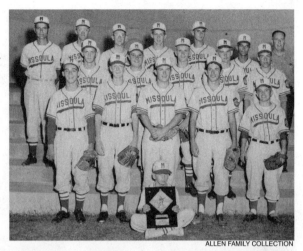

Middle row second right as a member of Missoula's American Legion state runner-up squad in 1958. Missoula gave Dave McNally and Billings a run for the state championship that summer.

ALLEN FAMILY COLLECTION

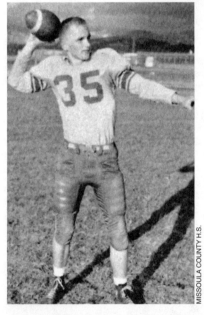

MISSOULA COUNTY H.S.

As a sophomore quarterback on the Missoula County High football team.

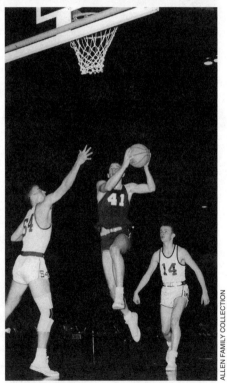

ALLEN FAMILY COLLECTION

Driving for two points during a varsity basketball game as a key performer for Missoula County High, which played for the state championship in 1959, '60 and '61.

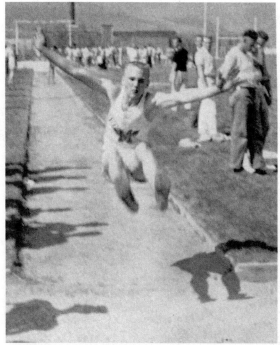

Competing in the long jump as a sophomore for the MCHS track team in 1959.

MISSOULA COUNTY H.S.

MISSOULA COUNTY H.S.

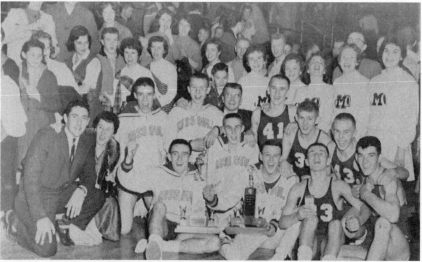

Number 41 celebrates the Spartans' 1959 state high school basketball championship with MCHS teammates, cheerleaders and fans. Head coach Lou "Rock" Rocheleau and his wife are at lower left.

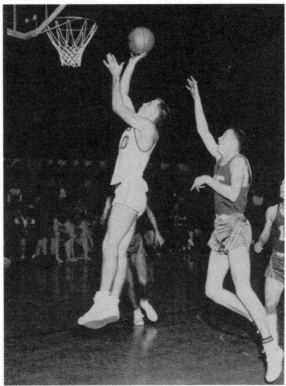

Shooting a layup as a junior all-state honorable mention performer in 1960.

MISSOULA COUNTY H.S.

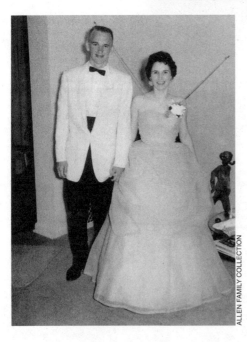

With Jackie Gordon on prom night, circa 1960.

ALLEN FAMILY COLLECTION

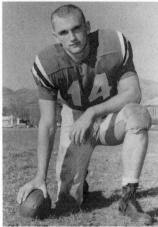

UNIVERSITY OF UTAH

As a freshman on the University of Utah football team.

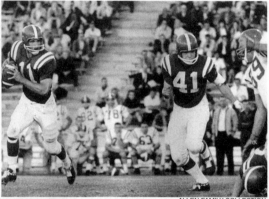

Running the Utah offense at quarterback. Number 11 played both QB and defensive back from 1962 to 1964 for the Utes.

ALLEN FAMILY COLLECTION

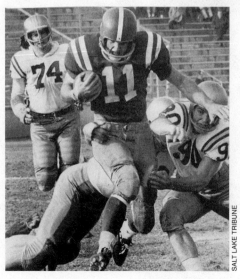

SALT LAKE TRIBUNE

Rushing for 12 yards against UCLA as a sophomore quarterback during the 1962 season. Bruin defenders are Al Geverink (90) and Randy Schwartz (74).

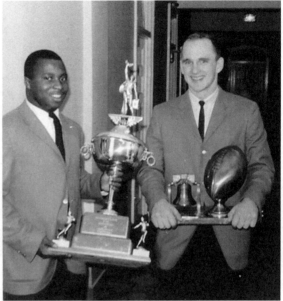

Holding the 1964 Liberty Bowl MVP trophy alongside Utah teammate Ron Coleman after leading the Utes to a 32-6 win over West Virginia.

ALLEN FAMILY COLLECTION

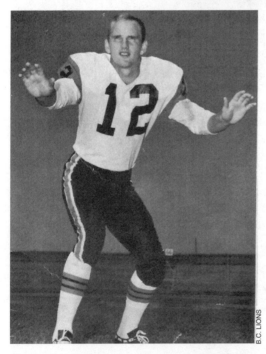

B.C. LIONS

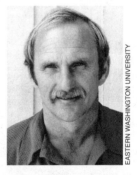

EASTERN WASHINGTON UNIVERSITY

An assistant coach at Eastern Washington in 1981.

As a rookie defensive back/quarterback in 1965 for the British Columbia Lions of the Canadian Football League.

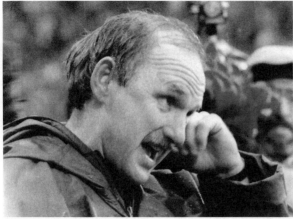

ALLEN FAMILY COLLECTION

Those were raindrops, not tears, during a Portland State game in the late 1980s.

PORTLAND STATE UNIVERSITY

Pacing the sidelines before a Portland State contest.

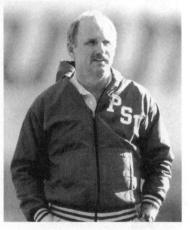

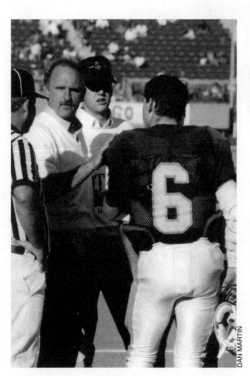

DAN MARTIN

Discussing the situation with an official and All-America quarterback Chris Crawford (6) during the 1988 season.

Aboard Tiki during a 1990 television promotion for PSU football tickets.

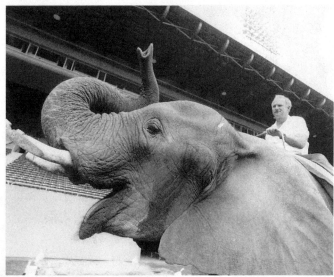

PORTLAND STATE UNIVERSITY

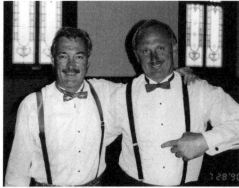

In church with best man Jerry Bradley before marrying Barbara Rigg on July 28, 1990.

ALLEN FAMILY COLLECTION

ALLEN FAMILY COLLECTION

With Barb in Portland.

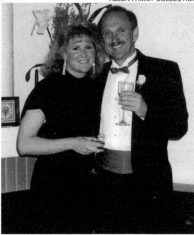

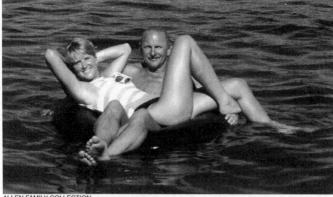

ALLEN FAMILY COLLECTION

Relaxing at Flathead Lake with Barb.

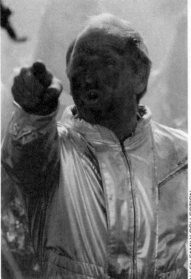

After being "shot" out of a cannon and declaring, "If you don't buy your season tickets this year, I'm gonna land in your backyard!" Yet another popular promotion at PSU.

ALLEN FAMILY COLLECTION

CHUCK SCHEER/BOISE STATE

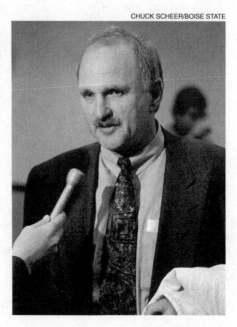

Conducting a media interview in Boise on December 9, 1992, after being named BSU's head football coach.

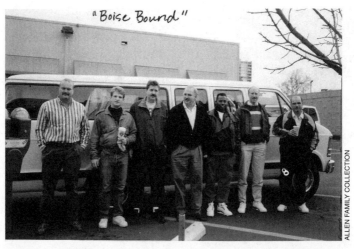

The new BSU coaches leaving Portland for their news jobs in Boise. From left: Dave Stromswold, Barry Sacks, Tom Mason, Pokey Allen, Ron Gould, Tom Osborne and Al Borges.

CHUCK SCHEER/BOISE STATE

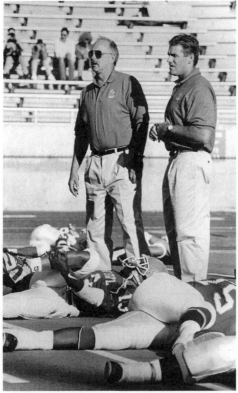

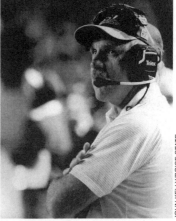

A worried look during a long and difficult 1993 season.

Surveying the situation with assistant coach Pete Kwiatkowski during pregame warm-ups in Bronco Stadium in 1994.

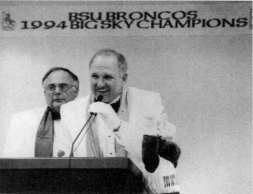

In formal attire at the weekly luncheon of the Bronco Athletic Association two days after beating Idaho for the Big Sky football championship in 1994.

JOHN KELLY/BOISE STATE

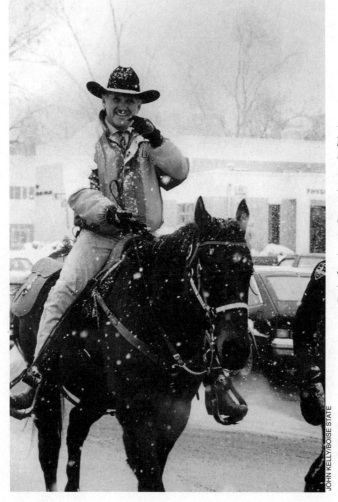

Keeping a promise to ride a horse down Boise's Broadway Avenue if more than 20,000 fans attended BSU's 1994 Division I-AA semifinal game against Marshall two days earlier.

JOHN KELLY/BOISE STATE

Portfolio

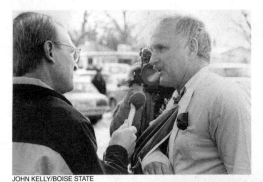

With arm in a sling following minor surgery, preparing to board the BSU football team's charter flight to Huntington, West Virginia, for the 1994 Division I-AA championship game. At the time, it wasn't known the problem was cancer.

Addressing the team in Marshall Stadium the night before the 1994 championship game against Youngstown State.

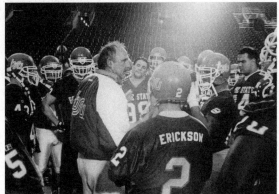

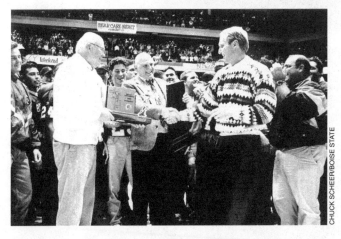

Showing the side effects of radiation treatment, accepting the Big Sky championship and national runner-up trophies from BSU president Charles Ruch (holding Big Sky trophy) and athletic director Gene Bleymaier (shaking hands) with jubilant players and coaches at halftime of a 1995 BSU basketball game.

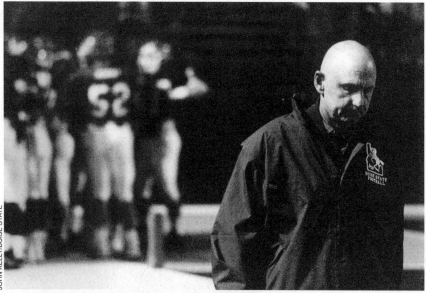

JOHN KELLY/BOISE STATE

Cancer, problems with the Idaho Statesman, *and a disappointing performance by the BSU football team made for a long season in 1995.*

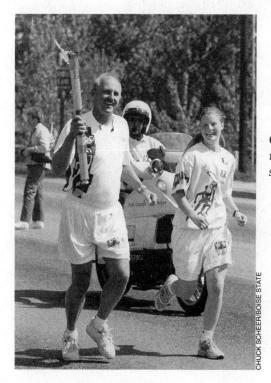

CHUCK SCHEER/BOISE STATE

Carrying the Olympic torch near the BSU campus in the spring of 1996.

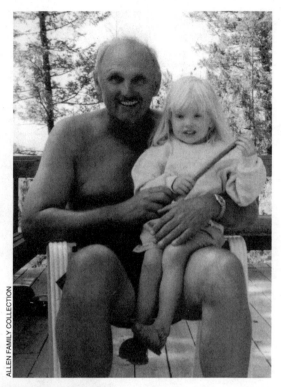

With daughter Taylor at Flathead Lake during the summer of 1996.

ALLEN FAMILY COLLECTION

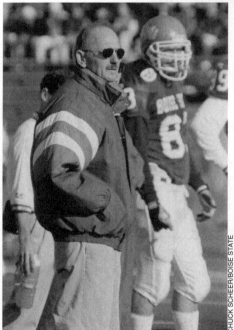

Idaho vs. BSU, November 23, 1996.

CHUCK SCHEER/BOISE STATE

Central Florida, Eastern New Mexico—anything with some kind of geographical identity to help us publicize the game." As expected, we got the invitation to the playoffs *and* the home-field advantage, but our first-round opponent didn't quite have the name recognition we had hoped for. I mean, *Mankato State*?

As it turned out, we didn't need any promotional gimmicks because our game with the Mavericks of Mankato, Minnesota, drew a Division II playoff record crowd of 19,363. (In Portland State annals, it was second only to the Civic Stadium crowd of 26,102 that witnessed the Oregon State-PSU game in 1983.) And those who showed up were treated to a classic. The Mavericks' wishbone offense piled up 287 yards on the ground, but we made some big plays, and with 5:40 remaining we appeared in pretty good shape with a 27-14 lead and in possession of the ball at the 50-yard line.

But then we fumbled, and Mankato State had new life when it recovered the ball on our 43. Led by quarterback Mike McDevitt, the Maverick offense hurriedly drove for a touchdown, cutting our lead to 27-21 with less than four minutes to go. To no one's surprise, Mankato State tried an onside kick on the ensuing play; much to our horror it worked as the Mavericks recovered the ball near midfield. Needing a TD and an extra point to pull out the win, McDevitt again directed his offense downfield, and with 35 seconds remaining the visitors had a first down on our 11-yard line. With staggering swiftness we were on the verge of a monumental collapse. But our defense stiffened; after a two-yard run and two incomplete passes Mankato State was faced with a fourth down on the nine-yard line in the closing seconds. McDevitt took the snap, faded back and threw a pass to halfback Jerome Tatum, who was running a curl pattern into the middle of the end zone. Cornerback Scott Laboy reached Tatum a split second after the ball did and was able rip the ball from Tatum's arms before he had possession; the pass was ruled incomplete with seven seconds to go. The Mankato State players and coaches were incensed, claiming Tatum had the ball long enough for the pass to be ruled complete, but the call stood. We dodged the proverbial bullet and were in the national semifinals. Our victory was tempered by some bad news, however: Delgardo had suffered a cracked shoulder blade.

With our dramatic victory, PSU football suddenly became a hot commodity in Portland. Things got even more exciting when we again got the nod for the home-field advantage in the semifinals the following week against Northern Michigan. Civic Stadium's capacity is 23,150, but with portable bleachers the number of seats can be expanded to more than

30,000. We knew it would cost the university money to have the bleachers installed, but we anticipated a record-breaking crowd, so our athletic department decided to have the extra seating put in.

Well, shoot, Mother Nature didn't cooperate; in a steady downpour we hosted NMU on December 5 for the right to play for the national championship. We still drew 17,795 fans, but I'm certain we would have pulled in 25,000 or more with decent weather. Again our defense was outstanding. The Wildcats scored a TD on their first possession with a 77-yard drive, but those were to be their only points of the game. Our defensive unit limited Northern Michigan to 219 yards total offense and forced four turnovers. We scored 13 first-half points on a touchdown run by fullback Tommie Johnson, who rushed for 111 yards, and two field goals by Mike Erickson. Then we relied on our defense in the second half. In the third quarter cornerback Dominique Hardeman intercepted a Northern Michigan pass, and safety Joe Rodgers had two picks in the final four minutes to help preserve the win as we advanced to the national championship game in Florence, Alabama.

Our opponent in the nationally televised Division II final on December 12 was Troy State of Alabama, the 1984 national champ and a semifinalist the previous year. The Trojans, who had defeated Central Florida 31-10 in the semis the previous week, featured a high-powered wishbone offense led by lightning-quick quarterback Mike Turk. I wouldn't say the Trojans had the home-field advantage, but they *were* only 300 miles from home. Still, I was in no position to complain since we got to host our first two playoff games.

We were all a bit nervous at the start of the title game; fortunately, our defense was outstanding in the first two quarters as we held a 10-3 halftime advantage. Troy State tied the game at 10 on Turk's one-yard touchdown run early in the second half, but we regained the lead at 17-10 on a 37-yard touchdown pass from Crawford to Corrigan with 9:28 to go in the third period. But Troy State took a 24-17 lead before the third quarter was over on a pair of reverses that went for touchdowns—49 yards by Titus Dixon and 15 yards by Greg Harris. Our players never quit, though. Midway through the fourth quarter our offense mounted a drive from our own 14-yard line. Crawford deftly directed our offense downfield, and when Tommie Johnson broke loose for a 40-yard run to the Troy State four-yard line, a game-tying score seemed imminent. But it was not to be; with 5:28 to go Troy State defensive back Doug Mims intercepted a Crawford pass at the Trojan goal line to thwart our bid. A few minutes later the Trojans iced the game with a 51-yard touchdown run by Turk for a 31-17 victory. Crawford completed 22 of 37 passes for 287 yards and Corrigan had eight catches for 141 yards, but our running game, with Delgardo playing hurt in a shoulder harness, could muster only 135 yards, and our defense simply couldn't contain the elusive Turk, who rushed for 175 of his play-off-record 190 yards in the second half.

We finished the year with an 11-2-1 record, the best in Portland State history. I was fortunate enough to receive league and district Coach of the Year honors. A couple of months later I was named winner of the 1987 Slats Gill Award at the 40th Banquet of Champions, an annual event that recognizes Oregon's top sports personalities. The Gill Award goes to the state's outstanding coach or administrator. Interestingly, the Prep Athlete of the Year award went to basketball player Trisha Stevens of Philomath, who eight years later would be named women's basketball coach at Boise State while I was the school's football coach.

OF COURSE, LOSING the national championship game hurt a great deal. But I'll tell you what: We had a great ride getting there. Football should be fun. Not only for the players, but for the coaches—especially the head coach. I mean, why be so serious? I did have one worry, however, as my second season at Portland State drew to a close: If we didn't continue to excel on the field, I thought people might be quick to dismiss the '87 season as a flash in the pan and lose interest. Sure, we had a great year, but college football is a fickle game and the enthusiasm and excitement we created could fade just as fast as it had materialized; I knew we had to keep the program in the public eye.

Using our appearance in the Division II national championship game as a springboard, we really got the football program rolling—on and off the field. I never really thought of myself as some kind of pitchman when we started to do our offbeat promotions at Portland State, but they seemed to work. Looking back, I think I developed some promotional know-how from people I had known long before I came to Portland. Three of my closest friends—Jerry Bradley, Mike Munsey and Ken Staninger—have flourished as businessmen because of their entrepreneurial spirit and ability to promote and market their particular product. Bradley is a prosperous stock promoter, Munsey owns a very popular restaurant, and Staninger is a successful real estate and sports agent. All three make their living by dint of personality, hard work and salesmanship, and some of their knowledge must have rubbed off on me over the years because I knew that selling *our* product—especially with our limited budget—required more than just putting a winning football team on the field every Saturday.

Not all our promotions were a huge success at first. But it wasn't from lack of trying. I mean, it was our *coaches* who first organized the tailgate parties that coincided with PSU home football games. It wasn't in our job description, but that's exactly what we did the first year or so. Often with Jerry Bradley's help, we would throw pregame and postgame parking-lot parties in an effort to generate interest in Viking football games. But like most of our other early promotional efforts, overcrowding was seldom a problem. Obviously, the other coaches and I couldn't attend the pregame gatherings, but I can recall more than a few postgame affairs that involved just Bradley, our coaching staff (we always made sure that Jerry saved us a few beers), a couple of other friends and a few transients off the street who joined us because we had free hot dogs.

But a year or so later, the vagrants were replaced by real live fans. Eventually there were an estimated 3,000 folks regularly going to PSU tailgate parties; people were actually planning their entire Saturday around our games. Sure, it was fun. But Viking football games didn't just become popular social events by themselves; the other coaches and I worked awfully hard to drum up community support.

One time we put together a booster/alumni/faculty party at a Beaverton watering hole called Chevys. One of the reasons we picked that particular establishment was because it served free hors d'oeuvres and seemed to attract good-looking women. We invited every professor at the university and had the Viking cheerleaders go out and put up some banners and invite everybody they could, but I don't think we had more than 25 people show up for our first party. But our social gatherings, like our football games and tailgate parties, began to grow in popularity. We did those things because I knew we couldn't consistently win football games without significant backing—both financially and in terms of attendance. We needed to put people in the stands and we needed to raise money. At a time when the Viking football program needed some new life breathed into it, I think I was at the right place at the right time for PSU. And in the process, I was earning a reputation as a coach who was a bit, well, different.

"Allen never apologized for letting the good times roll," the *Oregonian's* Ken Goe once wrote. In the same article, Goe quoted Al Borges regarding my personality: "Most of the powers that be have an image of the way a head football coach should appear in public," Borges said. "They feel he should be a straight-laced guy in a business suit who says the right things at the right time and, above all, always is to be taken seriously. Pokey doesn't fit that mold. That isn't his personality."

"In the stagnant world of college football, Allen is what you'd call a tornado of fresh air," commented *St. Louis Post-Dispatch* writer Tom Wheatley in *The Sporting News*. "Was Pokey born kooky, or was it an acquired trait?" My response? "I think it's been acquired since we got [to Portland]," I told Wheatley. "I've always been promotion-minded. And when I came here, the financial situation wasn't good. So we tried to create an atmosphere where people would have some fun."

It became even more fun when I brought Dream Weaver back to Portland in the fall of 1988. In January of that year PSU president Natale Sicuro appointed me interim athletic director to replace the departed Dave Coffey, who quit after citing "philosophical differences" with the university's administration. In my new capacity I hired Weaver as the athletic department's director of marketing and promotions. And Steve, who got his name from the mid-70s pop song "Dream Weaver," never met a promotion he didn't like.

Case in point: In December 1987 I appeared before Oregon's State Board of Higher Education during a presentation on the PSU campus to show that our program had enough support to consider moving up to Division I-AA. I hadn't prepared any formal remarks, and I kind of felt like I was being thrown to the wolves. Anyway, one of the board members looked at me real seriously and said something like, "Coach Allen, you know Portland State football has never really drawn that well. What makes you think the program is ready to move up to a higher division?" I really didn't know how to respond, so I blurted out something like, "I'll tell you what. I'll bet my paycheck that we can go Division I-AA, and we won't average 6,000 people, we'll average *10,000* people." Now, that was a pretty bold—some called it stupid—thing to say because Portland State had never come close to that figure. Excluding our two playoff games in 1987, PSU's average home attendance during the previous 10 years was less than 4,800, and the best single-season average was 8,612 in 1976.

It was a spur-of-the-moment statement that I didn't think anyone would remember—or take seriously. But in mid-October of 1988, more than halfway through the following football season, Bill Clunie, a columnist for the *Vanguard*, PSU's student newspaper, recalled the declaration I had made to the state board and used his column to bet his paycheck against mine. I remember walking into my office the day the edition of the *Vanguard* containing Clunie's piece came out; everybody in the athletic department was hopping mad—even the secretaries. Most of them thought Clunie was being a smart ass and trying to show me up, but Weaver and I saw it differently. "Hey," Dream said, "why don't we take him up on it?" So a few days later we held a press conference on the 50-yard line of Civic Stadium to announce the bet: Clunie would donate one month's pay, about $350, to the athletic department scholarship of my choice if the Vikings broke the 10,000 mark at the gate. If we didn't, I would forfeit one of my checks (about $2,100 after taxes and IRA payments) to the English department scholarship of Clunie's choice. "I forgot about the TV cameras [at the board meeting]," I joked. "I didn't mean it." But we made the bet anyway.

Now remember, our club was already seven games into the '88 season at the time, and with a 4-2-1 record we hardly looked like the world-beaters from the previous year. Moreover, our average attendance was just over 8,000 with just two home games remaining on the schedule. Most observers said it was a pretty dumb bet on my part—"I think we may be passing the hat around," Curtis Delgardo jokingly told the *Oregonian*—but our ace in the hole was our belief that we would make the Division II playoffs again, which would undoubtedly boost our gate figures. Weaver has a real ability to turn insignificant things like a column in a college newspaper into a major promotion, and all of a sudden the bet was a big deal in Portland. I remember walking down a street and some guy rolling down his car window and shouting, "I'm coming to the next game, Pokey! Don't worry, we're gonna save your paycheck!" I mean, it was crazy. Ever the promoter, Weaver even tried to contact the producers of *Late Night With David Letterman* to see if they had any interest in having some fun with the wager. They didn't, but the person in New York that Dream talked to did have one question: "Is his name *really* Pokey?"

Our next game was at home against Southern Utah, a 52-24 victory in which we amazingly drew 14,163. After road wins over Sacramento State and Cal Lutheran, our regular-season finale was at home against Montana on November 12, and the hoopla surrounding the bet was growing. G.I. Joe's and some other Portland businesses sponsored a large ad in the *Oregonian* that contained a picture of me and a coupon for our game against the Grizzlies. "PROTECT POKEY'S PAYCHECK," the ad blared in large block letters. "Use Your 'Pokey's Paycheck' Coupon & Save $2 Off Any Ticket to See Montana vs. Portland State. Let's Fill Civic Stadium So Pokey Won't Have to Pay!" At the bottom of the ad in small type was the following message: "In a public hearing before the State Board of Higher Education, coach Pokey Allen promised to give up his paycheck if this year's home-game attendance didn't average 10,000 fans. His bluff was called—13,700 fans at the Montana game will protect Pokey from losing his paycheck."

Well, our 21-0 win over the Grizzlies attracted 13,934. Next came three

Division II playoff contests in Civic Stadium that drew an average of 14,687. I won the bet and we won 10 straight games and earned a return trip to the national championship game in the process. My wager with Clunie drew plenty of media attention, including a story in the *Los Angeles Times*. "When it came time to collect on the bet, [Allen and Weaver] went soft. They didn't want to take Clunie's money," wrote *Times* reporter Scott Howard-Cooper. "They talked about holding a postseason tailgate party, making a cake to look like a check and having Clunie eat that. But no. Clunie paid up. And Pokey and Dream said they took the money. Others aren't so sure they didn't slip most of it back to him. Pokey just thinks about the attention it all got and smiles."

Did we take Clunie's money? Shoot no. But I sure enjoyed winning that wager.

That same article also noted that Portland State's average home attendance in 1988 was 11,594, a 285 percent increase at the gate since 1985—the year before our staff arrived.

I'd be lying if I said I wasn't enjoying the attention our program was getting. It really was a fun time at Portland State, and because of our success on the football field, I got to rub elbows with some pretty famous people—like Vice President George Bush, who would be elected president a couple of months after we met. On August 23, 1988, Bush was scheduled to speak at Pioneer Courthouse Square in downtown Portland during a stop on his presidential campaign tour. Along with about two dozen prominent Republicans, I got to meet the vice president and joined him on the platform in front of a crowd of more than 5,000 people. Just before the rally, Bush and I were introduced. As we shook hands I think I said something real deep and meaningful like, "Hey, how ya doin'?" Heady stuff, huh? But then, I've never been known as the world's greatest conversationalist. In any case, I got a note from Bush a month later thanking me for appearing with him at the rally. "Having you there meant a great deal to me," the note said. "Best of luck for a great season."

ABOUT THAT '88 season …

With 16 starters from our national runner-up squad coming back, another great year indeed seemed quite possible. Even so, the other coaches and I knew the 1987 season would be a tough act to follow. Even with talent, depth and great coaching, good fortune is a key ingredient to any successful season, and we knew we'd need our share of luck to continue in 1988 what we had started in '87.

Our returning players included Chris Crawford, Curtis Delgardo, Tim

Corrigan, Barry Naone and Dave Swanson on offense while the defense was led by ends Anthony Spears and Brent Napierkowski and linebacker Kevin Wolfolk. In a word, we were loaded. A couple of preseason publications even picked us as the No. 1 Division II team in the nation. But we also had what I thought was the toughest Division II schedule in America that year. In addition to hosting Division II powers Texas A&I and Indiana University of Pennsylvania, we also had games with Idaho, Eastern Washington and Montana of the Division I-AA Big Sky Conference. I know it's a cliché, but I think some of our players read too many preseason press clippings and started feeling too cocky for their own good. As it turned out, the other coaches and I had legitimate concerns because we got off to a lousy start.

We opened the season with a disappointing 31-31 deadlock in Spokane with EWU and my old boss, Eagles coach Dick Zornes, and then lost 27-18 to Keith Gilbertson's Idaho squad, which was ranked No. 1 among I-AA schools at the time, as Vandal star and future NFL quarterback John Friesz threw three TD passes. In the friendly confines of Civic Stadium we finally got our first win, a 21-3 triumph over Cal Poly-San Luis Obispo. But that was followed by a loss to a talent-laden Texas A&I team. With our club trailing 22-7 at halftime, Crawford, playing with a painful elbow injury, rallied our offense, tying the game at 22 late in the third quarter with an eight-yard TD pass to Corrigan and a two-point conversion to Delgardo. But the Javelinas scored late in the game to break the deadlock and post the 29-22 win. After four weeks we were spinning our wheels; what was supposed to be the best team in school history had stumbled out of the gate with a 1-2-1 record.

Our coaching staff was discouraged, to say the least. But you know what? Even during that difficult time we were still optimistic—and we were still having fun. In fact, I can still recall a pretty interesting scene at Portland's East Bank Saloon after the Texas A&I game. As is our current custom at Buster's in Boise, the other Viking coaches and I would usually unwind with a few beers at the East Bank Saloon following a home game. Whether we were there to celebrate or drown our sorrows, we would be joined by plenty of fans, sometimes numbering in the hundreds, who were also at the bar following the game. On that particular night we were feeling pretty low, but the place was hopping and we started mingling; Al Borges started singing with the karaoke, and we began to lighten up and have a few laughs. Like I've said, nobody hates losing more than I do, but I firmly believe that if you work hard and believe in yourself, good things are eventually going to happen.

Years later, some people referred to the accomplishments of our football programs at Portland and Boise as "magic." Magic my foot. It wasn't magic; it never has been. You know, when things get real tough, all you have to do is reach down way deep. You've got to work harder, you've got to stay focused, you've got to persevere, you've got to believe in yourself and in what you're doing. Then it's easy. Just sit back and wait for the "magic" to happen. So all that magic that people talk about, it wasn't magic. It was hard work, it was dedication, it was commitment, it was believing in the coaches and players whom I picked to support me. Our success is based on a group of dedicated coaches who can deal with adversity, who are willing to work all that much harder when things aren't going well, and who are committed to the success of the program. I had those kind of coaches at Portland State then and I have them at Boise State now. I mean, talented guys like Tom Mason, Dave Stromswold and Barry Sacks haven't stuck with me for more than 10 years out of blind loyalty. They believe in the same things I do. So when we were staring at that 1-2-1 record after the Texas A&I loss in September of 1988, we were concerned, but we didn't panic or overreact. We figured if we made the proper mental and physical adjustments we would turn things around. And we did.

Part of the reason for our slow start that year was a rash of injuries to key players, but I've always said excuses are for losers. After the Texas A&I game our killer schedule got easier, some of the players' bumps and bruises began healing, and our team got better.

With a 42-0 thrashing of Western Football Conference foe Santa Clara on October 1 we evened our overall mark at 2-2-1 and improved our league record to 2-0. The following week we hosted third-ranked Indiana University of Pennsylvania. Amazingly, we had only 32 yards total offense in the first two quarters and trailed 11-0 at halftime. For all intents and purposes, our season was slipping away. We were unranked and just a .500 team at the time; a loss would surely eliminate us from the playoff picture. Now, I'm not a real fire-and-brimstone type, but the other coaches and I had a few, um, choice words for our players at halftime. Fortunately, they responded as Crawford threw a pair of third-quarter touchdown passes for a 12-11 advantage. But the Indians shot ahead 17-12 with a TD early in the final period. Crawford, however, was his usual brilliant self as he directed a 76-yard drive in the fourth quarter, hitting Corrigan with a 15-yard touchdown pass to give us the hard-earned 20-17 win. That game was our wake-up call.

We beat Cal State-Northridge 45-13 the following week, which was followed by our 52-24 triumph over Southern Utah in the game that began my bet with the *Vanguard's* Bill Clunie. Meanwhile, we had climbed to the fifth spot in the Division II poll and regained our place among the nation's elite with a come-from-behind 43-29 victory over sixth-ranked Sac State to improve our record to 6-2-1. Our 49-0 win over Cal Lutheran the following week allowed us to finish unbeaten in league play for the second consecutive year, and our 21-0 triumph over Montana in our regular-season finale gave us an 8-2-1 overall mark.

Crawford was the runner-up for Division II Player of the Year award, and he and Naone earned All-America honors while 16 Portland State players were named to the All-WFC team. Delgardo broke his own single-season school rushing record with 1,251 yards, was fifth in the nation in scoring, and earned WFC Offensive Player of the Year honors while linebacker Kevin Wolfolk was named the league's Defensive Player of the Year. Our offense was ranked fifth nationally, and for the second straight season I was named both WFC and district Coach of the Year. In direct relation to our success on the field was this interesting financial statistic: fund raising at Portland State had increased fivefold. We were on a roll as we advanced to the Division II playoffs for the second year in a row.

Postseason awards are nice, but our goal was to capture what had barely eluded our grasp the previous season—the NCAA Division II national championship. Our climb back to the title game, however, would be even tougher this time around because the Division II playoff format had been expanded from eight to 16 teams, which meant we would need three wins instead of two to earn a return trip to Florence, Alabama.

Just like in 1987, our successful efforts to boost Portland State's attendance figures in 1988 were undoubtedly a key factor in the NCAA's decision to allow us to stay at home through the first three rounds of the playoffs. Aided by the drive to help save my paycheck, the Vikings' 1988 regular-season average attendance surpassed the 10,000-per-game mark, a figure the money-conscious NCAA could not ignore when making the '88 playoff pairings.

Our first-round visitor was Bowie State, which we dismantled 34-17. The Bulldogs of Bowie, Maryland, drew first blood with a first-quarter field goal, but then it was all Portland State as we scored 20 unanswered points en route to the victory. Our defense limited Bowie State to 216 total yards and Crawford threw a pair of touchdown passes as we advanced to the quarterfinals against Jacksonville State.

Crawford, who was ranked eighth in passing efficiency among the nation's Division II quarterbacks that year, showed why he was an All-America selection in our quarterfinal game against the Gamecocks of Jacksonville, Alabama. We held a 12-3 lead at the half, but Jacksonville State scored a touchdown in the third quarter and then took a 13-12 lead on a 17-yard field goal by Ashley Kay with 3:50 remaining in the game. Crawford then engineered an 84-yard drive and hit Corrigan with a 33-yard touchdown pass with 1:07 left, giving us an exciting 20-13 win. Crawford was brilliant. He passed for a career-high 375 yards, completing 27 of 41 passes and two TDs. Corrigan had eight catches for 168 yards. Our defense forced three turnovers and held the Gamecocks to 240 yards total offense.

Our come-from-behind victory set up a rematch with top-ranked Texas A&I, now called Texas A&M-Kingsville, in the semifinals. After having beaten us on our home turf 10 weeks earlier, the Javelinas were more than just a little perturbed that they had to return to Portland in the postseason. But our program simply had too many monetary enticements to dangle in front of the NCAA. First of all, Civic Stadium was one of the largest Division II facilities in the nation (PSU now plays in the Division I-AA Big Sky Conference), and our gate receipts and corporate backing allowed us to make an attractive bid to host the game and all but ensured a money-making venture. Also, because Civic Stadium is not on state property, the sale and consumption of beer in the facility is permissible.

Despite our home-field advantage, we knew we would have our hands full with Texas A&I. Not only were the Javelinas pissed off because they had to travel, they had a running-back tandem of *two* future NFL performers—Heath Sherman and All-American Johnny Bailey, a junior who had rushed for more than 1,400 yards during the regular season.

It would be hard to believe that Crawford could improve on his performance from the previous week, but he did against the Javelinas in front of 21,079 fans—the second-largest crowd in school history and an all-time Division II playoff record. Chris completed 25 of 32 passes for 270 yards and three touchdowns without throwing an interception. He hit Corrigan with a 14-yard TD pass for a 6-0 lead, but Texas A&I's vaunted running attack scored two long touchdowns, including a 55-yard dash by Bailey, for a 14-6 lead. But then Crawford took over with a brilliant second quarter. He directed a scoring drive that ended with Burnell Harvin's one-yard plunge, threw a 16-yard touchdown pass to wide receiver Greg Evers, and added an 11-yard TD throw to Delgardo, giving us a 28-14 advantage at the intermission. In the third quarter Ioasa Sione scored on a two-yard run to widen our lead to 35-14. Bailey scored a pair of fourth-quarter TDs for Texas A&I, but our lead was too big for the Javelinas to overcome and we advanced to the national championship game for the second straight year with a 35-27 victory, our 10th in a row. As our team triumphantly walked off the artificial turf at Civic Stadium, I thought back to the somber gathering at the East Bank Saloon 10 weeks earlier following our regular-season loss to the Javelinas. That night seemed like a long time ago now.

Unfortunately, our luck ran out once again in our return to Braley Stadium at the University of North Alabama in Florence. Our opponent in the championship game was North Dakota State, which was seeking its fourth national title in six years. The Bison, who downed Sacramento State 42-20 in the semis, featured a punishing ground game led by All-America running back Tony Satter. Crawford threw a pair of second-quarter touchdown passes—45 yards to Evers and a 16-yarder to Corrigan—as we battled NDSU to a 14-14 tie at the half. But the Bison wore our defense down in the second half and scored three unanswered touchdowns for a 35-14 lead. North Dakota State passed the ball only four times the entire game, but gained 339 yards on the ground. Our All-America passing duo of Crawford and Naone connected for an 11-yard TD late in the game to end their brilliant careers at Portland State, but it wasn't enough as we fell 35-21.

Needless to say, Florence isn't one of my favorite places to visit. With some breaks, we could have beaten North Dakota State. We didn't play our best game that day, but we played hard; that's all you can ask of your players. Still, I refused to let our back-to-back national championship losses drive me crazy. Well, not in the clinical sense anyway. How did I handle the bitter disappointment of losing two championship games in as many years? I think the *Oregonian's* Ken Goe did a good job in describing my "coping skills." In an interview with Crawford after Chris had finished school and left the program, Goe wrote the following: "Crawford remembers some of the Viking coaches and players gloomily sitting in a Florence establishment after [PSU's unsuccessful appearance] in the national title game. 'Coach Allen was in the corner, when all of a sudden he jumps up, rips off his jacket and goes sliding across the dance floor on his belly,' Crawford said. 'That's another thing you don't see from other head coaches. They don't teach you to "Gator." ... I don't know how you could have more fun with another coaching staff,' said Crawford, a former All-America quarterback at PSU. 'I start laughing just thinking about it.'"

Chapter 10

The Pride of PSU

In the summer of 1988, a few months after my breakup with Diane Rees, I started dating Barbara Rigg, a financial analyst for Pacific Corp. Credit and a fellow Montana native whom I would marry two years later. It was kind of interesting how we met. In 1985 I had introduced my friend Jerry Bradley to a Portland physical therapist named Sherri Niesen. Jerry and Sherri became romantically involved, and three years later I met Barb through Sherri—but it wasn't quite that simple. On the evening that we first met, Barb and I had dates with other people—sort of.

The story begins in Portland and an evening on the town with Jerry and Sherri, my date and me, and Barb. Barb, a close friend and former classmate of Sherri's at the University of Montana, had recently been transferred by her employer from Los Angeles to Portland. Because Barb was new in town, Sherri thought it would be a good idea for her to meet some new people, so we decided to get together at a jazz bar in downtown Portland and then have dinner at a nearby restaurant. Barb had a male friend visiting from Seattle, so the plan was for the six of us to meet at the bar. Well, Barb showed up, but her date didn't—which was fine with me because I was immediately attracted to her. So the five of us went out and had an enjoyable time. During the course of the evening, while my date was in the bathroom, I asked Barb out.

I was 45 and Barb was 27 when we met. Our age difference, however, was not an issue, and we really hit it off; after awhile she moved onto my houseboat, and marriage eventually followed. (Bradley and Niesen are no longer together but are still good friends, and both are playing a big role in my battle against cancer. As I work on this book in the fall of 1996, I'm living in Jerry's apartment in Vancouver while Sherri, who is doing her doctoral work on cancer research at the University of British Columbia, is helping me seek alternative treatments not available in the U.S.)

Thanks to my relationship with Barb, my personal life was great as 1988 came to a close. But I needed to make some changes professionally. In January 1989 I stepped down as Portland State's athletic director to concentrate on my head coaching duties. It was just too much being both football coach and AD. One problem was that the football offices and the athletic director's office were three blocks apart and I was spreading myself too thin. I also didn't care for the politics inherent in the AD's job. I was relieved to be rid of my administrative duties because I'm certain the football program would have suffered had I maintained my dual roles.

There were additional changes taking place among the Portland State hierarchy during that time. A couple of months before my resignation as AD, Natale Sicuro had been dismissed as the university's president and replaced on an interim basis by Roger Edgington, the school's executive vice president. It was decided that PSU's yet-to-be-named president should hire his or her own athletic director, so former AD Roy Love was asked to assume the newly created position of assistant to the president for athletics until the new administration was in office. In August 1990 Judith Ramaley was named PSU's president, and two years later assistant athletic director Randy Nordlof was promoted to AD. In my seven years at PSU there were four presidents, including Edgington, and four athletic directors, including me.

I try to steer clear of boardroom politics and bureaucratic wrangling, so I'm not entirely sure why there was such instability at Portland State during that period. Sicuro wasn't the easiest person to work with, which was part of the reason for his ouster by the State Board of Higher Education. But I never had any major problems with him, and in general he supported the football program. I mean, how could he not? We were creating a lot of excitement for the school and our players weren't causing any major problems. I figured as long as our team kept winning—and putting fannies in the seats—whoever was in charge would pretty much leave us alone. After all, I don't think it was an accident that PSU fund raising increased 500 percent after the 1988 football season. On the other hand, I don't mean to overstate or exaggerate the value of our program at Portland State—or any college football program for that matter. Of course academics are the primary function of any college, but let's face it: Few things can generate the exposure and community pride that a successful football program can.

And with back-to-back appearances in the Division II national championship game, Viking football was certainly in the limelight in Portland. Needless to say, our team's success was made possible by the hard work of many people, but as head coach, I was reaping the lion's share of the personal rewards. The NFL named me 1988 Small College Coach of the Year, and at Oregon's Banquet of Champions, I was named winner of the Slats Gill Award as the state's top coach for the second consecutive year. Started in 1957, the honor had previously gone to such outstanding coaches as Tommy Prothro, Dee Andros, Mouse Davis and Rich Brooks in football; Bill Bowerman in track; and Jack Ramsay and Ralph Miller in basketball. In fact, until my back-to-back awards in 1987 and '88, Oregon State's venerable Miller was the only repeat winner.

I felt very honored and considered myself in pretty select company when I accepted the award at the banquet from the Portland Trail Blazers' Clyde Drexler. But for me, the highlight of the evening was Chris Crawford's selection as the winner of the Bill Hayward Amateur Athlete of the Year Award. Out of 34 nominees the number of finalists had been pared to 11, which included Chris and Curtis Delgardo as well as Oregon State basketball star Gary Payton. It was pretty tough competition, but Chris had a great season—and career—at Portland State and he truly deserved the honor.

CRAWFORD TOPPED THE list of key players our program lost to graduation after the 1988 season, but he was by no means the only one. Also gone were wide receiver Tim Corrigan, tight end Barry Naone, center Dave Swanson, defensive ends Brent Napierkowski and Anthony Spears, linebacker Kevin Wolfolk and safety Joe Rodgers—stalwarts all. "The Vikings [are] faced with replacing most of the impact players who led them to consecutive appearances in the NCAA Division II championship game," wrote the *Oregonian's* Ken Goe. "On paper, [their] losses are staggering."

So what would it take to maintain our winning ways in 1989? Well, for one thing, we needed to keep the fans interested—and entertained. In that spirit we did another version of our television ad in which I menacingly stared into the camera and once again declared, "If you don't get your season tickets, a big meteor is gonna land in your backyard!" But we needed something more, something different, something … strange.

And strange is right up Steve Weaver's alley. Dream found that "something," and even Goe, who had become accustomed to our antics, seemed astounded. Six days before our 1989 season opener in Civic Stadium, Goe's article in the *Oregonian* revealed our newest promotional gimmick: "Believe it or not," he wrote, "when PSU opens the season on September 2 with a non-conference game against Cameron University, Allen is inviting the crowd to call his plays. Over the objections of offensive coordinator Al Borges, Allen has worked out a deal with G.I. Joe's in which the retail chain will pass out some sort of signaling device that will allow the fans to flash the PSU sideline whether they want to run or pass for one entire series."

We had a few critics who said we were making a mockery of the game and trying to imitate life beneath the big top. But that's ridiculous. If we had had a losing program, maybe *then* such criticism would have been valid. "This has been no carnival act," former *Oregonian* columnist Terry Frei once wrote in describing my approach to coaching. "I've never seen a more intense coach when that's appropriate." Frei was right. When things aren't going right, I can be an asshole with the best of them. But my basic approach to coaching is this: Football is a game and if you can't have fun playing a game, well, then when can you?

At halftime of our game against Cameron—a Division II team from Lawton, Oklahoma, that had a winning record the previous year—Weaver had a group of kids distribute 1,500 large white placards to the fans sitting in the two sections behind our bench. The cards, roughly the size of a record album cover, said RUN in large red letters on one side and PASS in green on the other. Based on a quick check of the cards being flashed, our gimmick required me to determine the majority and allow the fans to call our second series of offensive plays in the second half. We only had a 14-7 lead at the time, and the whole thing could have blown up in our faces.

Luckily, our second possession started on Cameron's 26-yard line after our defense recovered an Aggie fumble. As our offense took the field, it was a pretty crazy scene, which I think was best described by the *L.A. Times'* Scott Howard-Cooper: "This was perhaps the pinnacle of Portland State promotions," he wrote. "The crowd went wild. The scoreboard went wild, too, urging fans to 'Help Pokey Call the Play' and flashing 'Run' or 'Pass' underneath. The cheerleaders went wild, encouraging the fans to hold up their signs. The public-address announcer went semi-wild, telling the fans to help Pokey call the play. 'The place went absolutely nuts,' Weaver said. 'Pokey had a big grin on his face when he saw all the cards go up. It was a pretty amazing sight.' ... Without much time to get a quick reading and then send in the play, Pokey turned to his new 'offensive coordinators.'"

Now, the logical call is a run, but the majority of the fans held up their PASS signs, so I decided I better do as they said. You know, at that moment it didn't seem like such a great promotion. I mean, if we had screwed things up, we would have been the laughingstocks of college football. But junior quarterback Darren Del'Andrae completed a 14-yard pass, and a roughing-the-passer penalty moved the ball to Cameron's six. Then it really got crazy. I again turned around to see 1,500 frenzied fans holding up their cards and screaming at me. "Run!" some of them yelled. "Pass!" the others shrieked. I only had about 10 seconds to determine which group had the most signs and send in the play. It was close, but it looked like the "runs" had it. I conveyed the crowd's wishes to Borges, who signaled Del'Andrae, who called the play and handed the ball to Delgardo, who ran it in for a six-yard touchdown.

"Good thing, too," Howard-Cooper wrote. "If the fans had called for a pass, [Pokey] might have run anyway and claimed he had miscounted in the pressure of the moment. When Delgardo scored, the crowd was off the hook. So was Pokey."

Our stunt went nationwide following our 35-21 win over Cameron. In addition to the *L.A. Times'* account, *Sports Illustrated*, *The Sporting News*, the Associated Press and ESPN documented our card game with the fans. But that was just a once-a-season deal. Around that time Weaver also implemented another gimmick in which we would use one play submitted by a fan at each home game. Fans could submit their ideas by filling out forms at G.I. Joe's. The week before each home game, the other coaches and I would sort through the more than 100 mailed-in suggestions and select one play—preferably something on the tricky side—to use that Saturday. G.I. Joe's gave a $10 gift certificate for every yard the chosen play gained and $20 if it scored a touchdown. We usually employed the called-in play in the first quarter and I would wave a white towel over my head to let the crowd know that the selected play was about to be run.

Things were looking up at the start of the '89 season. Our victory over Cameron was followed by a 29-20 home triumph over Idaho and John Freisz, which marked Portland State's first-ever conquest of the Vandals in 11 tries. That win was especially gratifying because people were beginning to wonder if we were ever going to beat those guys from Moscow (a recurring lament my staff and I had to put up with not only in Portland but at our next coaching job in Boise). The loss dropped the Vandals to 0-2 under first-year coach John L. Smith (Keith Gilbertson had left UI the previous year to take the offensive coordinator's job at the University of Washington), but after their loss to us, Freisz and Company went on to win nine straight games and claim their third Big Sky title in a row.

AND THE PROMOTIONS just kept on coming. As an add-on to the PSU athletic department's annual Viking Classic fun run, the other coaches and I started a Pokey's Derby Team Challenge in which three members of our staff and I would race against other four-person teams in the 10-kilometer portion of the event. Teams that beat our average time would receive four tickets to the PSU home football game of their choice; teams that we out-performed would have to purchase four tickets at $9 each. Proceeds went to Portland State's track and cross country programs and the Viking Athletic Association Scholarship Fund. Another promotional effort was the football workshops for women that the other coaches and I conducted in an attempt to attract more female fans.

Also around that time, we began a weekly coach's radio show. It started off as a fairly predictable 30-minute production in which I looked back at the previous week's game and discussed our upcoming opponent. But when Weaver later took over as co-host … well, things got a little more off-the-wall. One thing we did was expand the show to an hour and add offensive coordinator Al Borges and defensive coordinator Tom Mason to the program. Every Thursday evening during the football season, we would broadcast from a local watering hole, knock back a couple of cold ones, and talk Viking football with callers and fans in the bar. We started doing the show at the East Bank Saloon, moved to Champions (the lounge in the Portland Marriott) in 1989, and later broadcast from various bars on a rotating basis.

I'll say this for Weaver—there was never a lull in the conversation. In fact, he has a tendency to dominate a discussion. I remember one time while we were on the air at Champions, Dream went off on a tangent about something and wouldn't shut up. So after a couple of minutes when it looked like he wasn't going to get off the subject anytime soon, I took off my headset, got up from my chair, walked to a pay phone in the lobby and "called in" to get back into the discussion and tell Dream to move on to the next topic. Coaches' shows can be pretty humdrum and routine, but that was hardly the case with Dream. Doing oddball stuff like that made the show interesting and great fun for the participants.

Weaver, who is now a sports talk-show host in Portland, was non-stop in everything he did. When he was working at Portland State I would see him in the morning and I usually never saw him again the rest of the day. He was out hustling, promoting, getting things done. You can often tell when real estate agents aren't doing well by the amount of time they spend in their offices. It's the same thing with a marketing/promotions guy. You never want to see him; he should be out schmoozing and glad-handing, and Dream did it well.

Lord knows how Weaver came up with some of his wacky ideas. I think it started in the mid-70s when he spent several days with master promoter and Chicago White Sox owner Bill Veeck. Dream, who was about 24 and director of public relations for the St. Louis Stars of the North American Soccer League at the time, sent Veeck a letter after reading his autobiography. Veeck wrote back, wishing Dream good luck in his promotional efforts and inviting him to "stop by" if he was ever in Chicago. Now, Dream is a pretty impulsive character; he took Veeck up on his offer and headed for Chicago the next day, driving straight to the White Sox owner's office at Comiskey Park. "Who are you?" Veeck asked when Dream showed up unannounced. "I'm Steve Weaver ... Remember?" Dream replied. "St. Louis Stars? ... Promotions? ... Your letter? ... You told me to stop by if I was ever in Chicago. Well, here I am." Veeck was dumbfounded. "Well, I wasn't expecting you to show up the same week, for chrissakes!" But Veeck took Weaver under his wing, and Dream actually ended up staying at his home for about a week, learning all he could from the king of sports publicity stunts.

With Dream's fertile (or was it deranged?) mind regularly coming up with some new plan, I continued to deliver speeches, make public appearances and do all kinds of publicity stunts and television promotions to help sell Portland State football. Throughout my coaching career, I have also helped almost all of the charities and worthy causes that have solicited my assistance. I don't know if I'd go so far as to say I had reached folk-hero status, but some people thought so. In September 1996 the *Oregonian's* Paul Buker visited me in Vancouver, British Columbia, to write an article about my battle with cancer. As he recounted my seven years at Portland State in the story, Buker said I "became a pop culture icon through a highly popular promotional campaign ... burned up, blown up and planted atop an elephant, pulling in record crowds at Civic Stadium."

Hey, I was just having fun. But by the late 1980s, I guess I had become somewhat of a celebrity in Portland. I feel a bit uncomfortable talking about myself, but I'd have to say that my accessibility and what's been described as an "aw-shucks charm" made me a media darling during those years. The way I come across in public, however, has never been a put-on; my unassuming public manner is the real deal because if there's one kind of person I can't stand, it's a phony. I suppose my personality *did* play a role in our football team's popularity, but that was just a small part of it. I think our program simply found a niche in Portland. The Trail Blazers were, and are, a big deal there, and Oregon and Oregon State football also draw well. But Blazer tickets are pretty expensive and hard to come by. As far as Oregon and OSU? I know a lot of people say, "Wow, Pac-10 football!" But I say big deal. I've seen some awful bad Pac-10 teams, and it's not like the two Oregon schools are perennial contenders for the league title. I was never preoccupied with competing against the Ducks and Beavers when I was at Portland State. My philosophy has always been simply to win as many football games as possible and have some fun doing it.

As an alternative to the Blazers and Oregon and OSU football, Viking football was a way for the average fan to have some fun and watch some relatively inexpensive and entertaining athletic competition. The games were fun and Civic Stadium is an outstanding facility. That's not to say PSU football wasn't entertaining before we showed up. From 1975 through 1980 Mouse Davis had a winning season every year except one, and his run-and-shoot offense made for high-scoring contests. But in the late 1980s and early '90s our entertaining brand of football combined with our goofy publicity stunts helped make Civic Stadium *the* place to be on Saturday evenings in the fall. In a word, we had become trendy.

I think Terry Frei put it best in a column he wrote in the *Oregonian* in 1990: "A few years ago, the following was inconceivable: On a Saturday when both Oregon and Oregon State played at home, the state's showcase game was in Portland. And Portland State ... outdrew OSU. The standards of evaluation have changed during Pokey Allen's coaching tenure. ... The Vikings have taken another step. They've extended their drawing power and their ability to catch your attention to the regular season. ... No longer is this the good-time team you pick up just in time for the NCAA Division II playoffs, after the Ducks' and Beavers' seasons are over.

"PSU football isn't life and death; it's fun and games. The PSU atmosphere remains reminiscent of a tailgate party, spilling into the seats. ... And PSU football, while a notch below what you could see in Eugene or (probably) Corvallis, is about the best that can be produced with a 40-scholarship limit, or less than half of what the Pac-10 schools offer."

I loved living in Portland and coaching at Portland State. From my perspective, Portland had all the ingredients necessary to produce a perennial winner. I've always believed that if you have a metropolitan area for a solid fan base, a nearby airport for recruiting and promotional trips, and the right people working with and for you, you can—with plenty of hard work—build and maintain a winning college football program.

I'm a gregarious person by nature, which made it easy for me to promote our program in Portland. I've always felt at ease in most social situations; it doesn't matter if I'm with bankers or hard hats. The weekly routine I followed when visiting my favorite haunts serves as an example. On Wednesdays a few colleagues and I would usually go to a hole-in-the-wall called Slammers Tavern for tacos and beer. On Thursdays during the football season we would broadcast our radio show at Champions or some other local bar; during the off-season Thursday was my night to visit Jake's and schmooze with prominent businessmen and other influential types. On Saturdays after home games we'd hit the East Bank Saloon and party with dozens of Viking football fans, and later move on to Champions for dancing. It really doesn't matter who I'm with, I just like being with people.

I think I can mingle with just about any group because I'm not awed by wealth and power. To be sure, a college football coach's duties include fund raising and networking with financial backers, but I've never been that hung up on money personally. When it comes to wealth and influence, I've experienced firsthand both ends of the spectrum—and everything in between. I come from humble beginnings, I enjoyed a modicum of personal wealth during one point in my life, and I've weathered the hardships and uncertainty of unemployment and financial insecurity. In my line of work I've met plenty of high rollers and well-to-do people— CEOs, bank presidents, business owners—in Portland, Boise and other places. For the most part, they're every bit like the rest of us—good, solid, down-to-earth people who work hard for what they have. During my years at PSU some of the best friends I made were among Portland's most affluent—company presidents like Jerry Nudelman, Bubby Cronin, Jack Garrison, Norm Daniels and Ron Schiff. What made these men stand out was that they didn't try to stand out.

I think it's that attitude that prompted the *Oregonian's* Ken Goe to write that I was probably "PSU's most popular fund-raising tool." Bob Tayler, the Viking Athletic Association's development officer at the time, once told Goe that he had taken me to everything from union meetings to country clubs. "Wherever [Pokey] goes," Tayler said, "he fits in."

HOWEVER, ON A few occasions it became evident that I needed to spend more time coaching and less time hobnobbing—following our loss to Montana in 1989, for instance. After our wins over Cameron and Idaho, we traveled to Missoula and lost to the Grizzlies in an afternoon contest 30-21. It was a bitter setback, compounded by the loss of perhaps our most important player—Curtis Delgardo, who suffered a broken leg in the second quarter. I was scheduled to catch a flight back to Portland to attend an important PSU fund-raising banquet and auction that evening while the rest of the team was to make the 600-mile return trip by bus.

But as I hurried out of the locker room to catch my flight, something just didn't feel right. In an article by Jack D. Welch in Portland's *This Week Magazine*, Weaver recalled the scene: "When [Pokey] came out of the stadium, the guys were all set to leave. They were beat up; their star's leg was broken; they were defeated physically and thoroughly. Pokey took one look at them and said, 'Call the school. Tell 'em I can't make it. … I'm taking the bus home, too.'"

With Delgardo out for the year, we were routed by Johnny Bailey and Texas A&I 31-12 in Kingsville the following week and fell to 2-2; suddenly, things weren't so promising. To make matters worse, Delgardo was just one of several starters to be felled by an injury that season. Early in the campaign our defensive line was beset by a rash of injuries, which no doubt had something to do with our sluggish start. On offense, running back Burnell Harvin picked up where Delgardo left off and rushed for over 100 yards in six straight games. But he, too, went down with a knee injury in our 42-19 win over Sacramento State in the ninth week. Other key players lost to injury in the second half of the year included All-America guard Bill Duarte, tackle Bob Dodd, tight end Ted Popson and middle linebacker Scott Taube. Needless to say, we struggled. But we somehow continued to win.

One reason was because of our quarterback, JC transfer Darren Del'Andrae. I thought Chris Crawford would be tough to replace, but Del'Andrae blossomed into one of the nation's top Division II quarterbacks and was a first-team All-America selection that year. With Harvin running and Duarte blocking (before they got hurt) and wide receiver Rinaldo Shackelford hauling in 48 passes for 1,082 yards and 10 touchdowns, Al Borges' offense was as explosive as ever during the regular season with Del'Andrae at the controls. We won six out of our final seven regular-season games to finish with an 8-3 overall mark and claimed our third straight Western Football Conference crown with a 4-1 record.

Del'Andrae was second in the nation in total offense with 265 yards per game, second in yards passing with 3,016 and fifth in passing efficiency. As a team we were second among the nation's Division II schools in passing with 282 yards per game, sixth in total offense with 446 yards and 17th in scoring with an average of 29.5 points per game. Harvin did an outstanding job picking up the slack for Delgardo, finishing 13th in the nation in rushing with an average of 108 yards a game. I was again named WFC Coach of the Year. For the fourth straight season we also boosted our numbers at the gate, pulling in an average of 10,246 fans per game, an increase of 251 percent from the year before our arrival. And fund raising was still up 500 percent from the '85 campaign. Then there was the most important accomplishment of the 1989 season: We were in the Division II playoffs for the third straight year.

We had some pretty high-scoring, action-filled affairs during our seven years at Portland State, but our first-round playoff contest in Civic Stadium against West Chester State College of Pennsylvania on November 18 was perhaps the greatest game in Viking football history. If nothing else, it was one of the most entertaining with a playoff-record 106 points lighting up the scoreboard. Del'Andrae threw for 381 yards and a playoff-record six touchdowns; tight end John Miller had 11 receptions for 159 yards and two touchdowns; and junior fullback Don Finkbonner, playing in the place of the injured Harvin, scored a record five TDs, rushed for 112 yards and caught 12 passes for 122 yards as we outlasted the Golden Rams 56-50 in a memorable overtime struggle. After battling to a 36-36 tie at the end of regulation, both teams scored a touchdown and a conversion in each of the first two extra periods and remained deadlocked at 50-50. In the third OT our defense prevented West Chester from scoring and Finkbonner settled matters with a one-yard touchdown run to mercifully end the three-hour, 38-minute marathon. "Do we have to play another game [next week]?" I joked to the media afterward. "Can we get a bye? We've played two games today."

My words proved prophetic; the slew of injuries we had suffered throughout the season and our exhausting win over West Chester took their toll and we just didn't have the horses or the energy the following week in the quarterfinals against another Pennsylvania opponent—Indiana University. After piling up 56 points the previous week, our offense sputtered and committed seven turnovers in a pouring rain and we lost to the Indians at home 17-0. Despite the inclement weather, the game drew 15,351 fans. Unfortunately, they had little to cheer about as we could muster only 294 yards total offense against IUP's outstanding defensive squad. It was the first time we had been shut out in 43 games.

GIVEN PSU'S 37-14-2 record and three straight playoff appearances in my four years as Viking coach, my name was occasionally bandied about when a head coaching position at another school opened up. In fact, in the same issue of the *Oregonian* that chronicled our playoff loss to IUP—November 26, 1989—Terry Frei wrote a column that bore the headline "Will Pokey find greener pastures?" In the article Frei surmised that I might be headed for a new job if the conditions were right: "This is a football coach we keep expecting to be out the door—but on his own volition, heading off to a Division I job. Somewhere along the line, somebody in a position of power at a program like Nevada-Las Vegas, New Mexico or Utah is going to say there's nothing wrong with going after a Division II head coach. He came to the PSU job talking of potential. Much of it has been realized, from lining up increasing corporate sponsorship and support, to putting good-time fans in the seats. ... PSU's first athletic priority should be to try to make Allen happy—and less inclined to listen to another offer."

There was some truth to Frei's words. A couple of weeks later I was one of six finalists for the head coaching job at Nevada-Las Vegas of the Division I Big West Conference. I eventually took myself out of the running because I didn't think UNLV had the facilities necessary to be competitive. Had I remained a candidate, I think I would have had a good shot at the job, which eventually went to Notre Dame assistant Jim Strong.

During that same period, I was offered the head coaching position with the Canadian Football League's Calgary club. Norm Kwong, the Stampeders' general manager, made me a pretty good offer, but the league was pretty shaky at the time, which was nothing new. Besides, we were having too much fun in Portland. After I turned down Kwong's offer, Wally Buono, who played his college football at Idaho State, was named Calgary's head coach in January 1990.

A year later I was one of two finalists for another CFL head coaching position. Hugh Campbell, my former boss with the L.A. Express and now the general manager at Edmonton, interviewed me for the Eskimos' head coaching job following the 1990 season. Hugh and I met in Canada and had a nice conversation, but he wasn't quite ready to offer me the position and I wasn't ready to take it. A couple of weeks later I took myself out of the running, and in February 1991 the job went to Ron Lancaster, the Eskimos' current coach.

I was rumored to be in the running for two other Division I head coaching positions, but I was never seriously considered for either of them. "The suspicion lingers that Allen's irreverence disqualified him from Division I jobs at Utah, his alma mater [in 1989], and Oregon State," wrote the *Oregonian's* Ken Goe. "He openly expressed interest in both and politely got the cold shoulder from both."

In the case of Oregon State, I guess they figured you're not supposed to have fun playing and coaching "major" college football. When Dave Kragthorpe vacated the OSU head coaching position after the 1990 season, there seemed to be a lot of people, including Frei, who thought the Beavers should give me a serious look. In the November 25 edition of the *Oregonian*, the headline atop his column read: "Pokey Allen belongs at the top of OSU's list." In the article Frei stated that "going into the interviews, the job should be Allen's to lose." At the time, however, Frei and others didn't know OSU wouldn't even give me the time of day.

"He knows Oregon," Frei wrote. "He's recruited the state. ... G.I. Joe's and PayLess Drug Stores have become major donors and sponsors, both because of Allen's direct efforts and the enthusiasm his program has generated. And, absolutely, Allen and his surprisingly stable staff can coach.

"Pretty soon [after 1986], the Vikings were putting customers in the seats, putting on entertaining shows and building up a constituency of fans who adopted Allen's team. ... Frankly, I—and a lot of people in the football business—thought he'd be out of PSU by now. But he's stayed in Portland because of two things: 1) He likes Oregon and wouldn't leave for just any job; and 2) The powers that be at programs that would represent a big step up for him can't get past this 'Division II' label and haven't given him a call. OSU shouldn't fall into the same trap. The Beavers should have Allen at the top of the list."

Frei was right on both counts. First, I was in no big hurry to leave Portland; it was going to take a pretty sweet deal at a bigger school to lure me from PSU. In fact, the only two college coaching jobs I formally applied for while at Portland State were UNLV in 1989 and Boise State in 1992. Second, I think there is a certain arrogance among Division I schools directed toward Division II programs. It was much the same in the USFL, which was looked upon scornfully by the NFL.

I think the Portland media and Viking boosters may have enjoyed stirring things up by drawing comparisons between the popularity of our program and that of Oregon and Oregon State. But there wasn't any bad blood between the coaching staffs. I got along well with the coaches from those schools. Former Oregon coach Rich Brooks always treated me well, and so did the coaches at OSU. If there was any resentment toward our program because of the media attention we got, I never experienced it first-hand. Besides, with the exception of our two trips to the national championship game, I don't think the *Oregonian* or Portland's radio and TV stations gave us any more coverage than they did the Beavers and Ducks. Well ... not a whole lot more. But I guess if *I* were a coach at one of those two schools, it might have bugged me somewhat to see some Division II school enjoying all this success and getting all this attention. Really, though, it's an apples and oranges thing. They were from the mighty Pac-10 and we were Division II. If we would have met Oregon or OSU on the field, they obviously would have beaten us soundly. Still, I think maybe some of our better teams might have been able to make it respectable.

AS OUR COACHING staff prepared for our team's 1990 spring drills, an amusing article appeared in the April 14 issue of the *Oregonian*. "The biggest news out of Portland State this spring doesn't have anything to do with red-hot quarterback prospects, injured running backs, or trips to the Division II national championship game," reported Paul Buker. "The bombshell dropped in the Parks Blocks recently concerned coach Pokey Allen. Long one of Portland's most eligible bachelors, Allen plans to get married in July to Barbara Rigg, a financial analyst from Great Falls, Montana."

Three and a half months later—on July 28, 1990—Barb and I got married in a Portland church. One of our wedding gifts was my MVP trophy from the 1964 Liberty Bowl, which I had lost track of several years earlier. Before then, the last time I remember seeing the trophy was around 1981 in the backseat of the car of a former girlfriend. Some of my buddies hunted it down, polished it up, and presented it to me at the reception.

A couple of weeks after the wedding, double sessions began, which marked the start of my fifth year as Portland State's coach. New Astro Turf had been installed in Civic Stadium during the off-season, which inspired Steve Weaver to come up with the slogan "The Greatest Show on Turf." Dream also decided that we needed to add a new wrinkle to our "meteor" television spot that year. After all, it had become a much-anticipated media event, and we didn't want to disappoint anyone. In an effort to top our previous season-ticket promotion, Weaver suggested that I ride an elephant in Civic Stadium for the TV commercial. "Hey, people say this program is run in a circus atmosphere anyway," he joked, "so why not an elephant?"

Needless to say, Dream knew just where to find such a beast in Oregon, so we rented a female elephant named Tiki from Wildlife Safari, a drive-thru wildlife park in Winston, Oregon, for $5,000. I found the price to rent Tiki a bit ironic. From what I recall, $5,000 was our original recruiting budget, and now we were renting *elephants* for $5,000. Anyway, with the cameras running I warily climbed atop Tiki, held on for dear life and hollered, "If you don't order your PSU season tickets now, a giant meteor *and* an elephant will land in your backyard!"

We had good reason to be lighthearted as the 1990 season drew near. Ticket sales were up, we were ranked sixth nationally in one preseason poll, and Curtis Delgardo was back after recovering from his broken leg the previous year. Moreover, All-America quarterback Darren Del'Andrae and linebacker Tim Upshaw, our most valuable defensive player from the '89 season, were also among our returning players.

In front of 14,222 fans, the second-largest season-opening crowd in school history, we kicked off the year with a 30-0 rout of Slippery Rock. Early in the second half we reintroduced our gimmick in which 1,500 fans sitting behind the PSU bench would call one series of offensive plays with color-coded cards. As he had done the previous year, offensive coordinator Al Borges threatened to resign (in jest, I think) if we did the stunt again. But we did it anyway. This time, however, things got kind of hairy because our series, designated in advance, began on our own two-yard line. "Oh, great, Pokey. This is just great," a sarcastic Borges said as the offensive unit took the field. "Nice goddam going. You're gonna have the fans call the goddam plays from the goddam two-yard line. This makes a lot of goddam sense."

I was afraid to look into the stands, but I knew I had to. Borges shook his head in disgust. Then he began to grin, evidently enjoying my predicament. To my dismay (but not to my surprise), the majority of our so-called offensive coordinators held up their PASS placards. Borges couldn't help but look at me with an I-told-you-so expression on his face. I don't think he would have been so smug if we hadn't had a 23-0 lead. "Al," I said, "we've got problems here." "No shit," he replied. Despite the fans' directive, I called a running play, in which Don Finkbonner gained three yards. A few boos, obviously directed at me, floated down from the stands. "Al," I said to Borges as the players unpiled and returned to the huddle, "run the goddam ball. I won't even look in the stands." Del'Andrae ran a keeper for no gain. More boos. "Ohmigod, Al!" I said. "We're in trouble!" Feigning horror, Borges whacked the sides of his face with his palms. "*Really?*" he said in mock surprise. The boos grew louder. Luckily, a face-mask penalty against Slippery Rock gave us a first down at the 20.

Once again, the majority of the fans flashed their green PASS cards. This time I acquiesced. Del'Andrae faded back and tossed a floater that was almost intercepted. The boos increased. "I told you this stupid gimmick of yours wouldn't work," Borges said half sneering, half laughing. Del'Andrae threw two more incompletions and we punted—and the booing continued. Now Borges was laughing. That was the beginning of the end of that deal. We tried it one more time in 1991, but it was just too risky.

Our season-opening win was followed by two more impressive home victories, 40-3 over Iowa Wesleyan in which Delgardo scored four first-half TDs, and 14-9 over Texas A&I, which drew a crowd of 17,798. But then we started to struggle, dropping three of the four league games that followed. Delgardo played well, but by the sixth game we had lost both Del'Andrae (rotator cuff) and Upshaw (knee) to season-ending injuries. The most frustrating period came in the middle of the season when we lost back-to-back games to Cal State-Northridge 19-18 and Santa Clara 28-26. After those two setbacks we split our final four games to finish third in the WFC with a 2-3 mark and 6-5 overall; we had been out of the playoff picture long before the season ended.

Still, we had a few bright spots that year. Delgardo concluded his brilliant career by winning his third league rushing title with 1,408 yards, and his average of 128 yards rushing per game was the sixth-best in the nation that year. At the conclusion of the 1990 season, Curtis stood sixth in NCAA history—in all divisions—with 6,942 all-purpose career yards. He broke every PSU rushing record and scored 54 touchdowns. Quarterback Don Bailey, who is now an assistant coach with me at Boise State, did an outstanding job after Del'Andrae got hurt. Despite starting only six games, Bailey passed for 1,629 yards and 10 TDs and completed 67 percent of his passes—fifth best in the nation—and broke Chris Crawford's single-season school record for passing accuracy. And despite our disappointing performance on the field, we set an all-time record at the gate with an average of 12,039 fans per game.

IN 1991 WE returned to our winning ways—and, of course, to Cap Hedges' oddball television commercials. Only this time some special effects were added to our TV spot. Part animated, part live, the commercial simulated me being blasted from a cannon on a large battleship (ostensibly in the Willamette River) high into the sky above Mount Hood. I then soared over Portland's Fremont Bridge and plummeted into Civic Stadium. Then the live portion of the commercial showed me rising from a cloud of smoke on the stadium's turf in front of some startled Viking cheerleaders. Dressed in a silver space suit with my face blackened and my body smoldering, I bounced up, walked toward the camera, pointed at it and declared, "If you don't buy your season tickets this year, *I'm* gonna land in your backyard!" It certainly didn't rival a *Star Wars* production, but like all the other commercials, it was a lot of fun to do.

During the preseason drills that year, redshirt freshman Matt James and junior college transfer John Charles had battled for the starting quarterback assignment. James got the nod, but our offense was ineffective in our season opener at home against 16th-ranked Mankato State. We could manage only 154 yards total offense and were held to minus-one yard rushing as the Mavericks beat us 10-7. We outscored Missouri Southern 56-38 at home the following week, but then lost to our old nemesis Texas A&I 35-14 to drop to 1-2.

In an effort to turn things around, the other coaches and I began to put in extra hours; consequently we dined heavily on fast food as we prepared for our next game against Sonoma State. The Monday and Tuesday preceding our game with the Cossacks, defensive line coach Barry Sacks and I had lunch at a nearby restaurant called Viking Burger. The connotation of its name to the contrary, Viking Burger served Malaysian food. (I think it had been purchased by Asian owners who decided to keep the name.) On both occasions, I ordered chow mein sauté with hot peanut sauce. Some of the other coaches and I also had pizza with anchovies on Tuesday night, and we made our regular stop at Slammers for beer and tacos on Wednesday evening.

In our game with Sonoma State that Saturday evening, we were holding a 9-6 lead in the third quarter when James broke his collarbone and was lost for the season. Charles stepped in and guided three second-half scoring drives as we pulled away for a 30-6 win. That was the start of Charles' starring role at PSU—and a steady diet of Malaysian food and pizza with anchovies for me.

I didn't really expect my eating habits to be of interest to the local media. But when we began a lengthy winning streak that coincided with my mealtime schedule, well, the Portland press thought it was newsworthy. "The next week [following the Sonoma State win], Allen dutifully ate the same fare on the same days at the same times at the same establishments, and PSU edged Southern Utah 33-30," wrote the *Oregonian's* Ken Goe. "Charles threw three touchdown passes and the Vikings made a late fourth-quarter, goal-line stand to preserve the win. So Allen made the rounds again the following week and PSU roared back from a 20-7 halftime deficit to thump Division I-AA Eastern Washington 35-23. Allen knew he was on to something."

I guess Goe was right. Led by Charles and a trio of first-team All-Americans—defensive back James Fuller, offensive tackle Larry Hall and tight end Ed Yoder—we won a school-record eight straight regular-season games to finish 5-0 in the Western Football Conference and 9-2 overall. In our 55-35 triumph over Cal Poly-San Luis Obispo in our regular-season finale, Charles erased a 22-year-old Division II record with 592 yards passing. In that game he threw a WFC-record eight touchdown passes, five to tight end Mike Palomino, and completed 28 of his 41 attempts. For the fourth time in five years we were league champs and in the Division II playoffs. "That means an NCAA record for consumption of peanut sauce, anchovies and tacos by a college head football coach," Goe wrote.

I'm not superstitious, but I do have a tendency to follow the same schedule when things are going well. During another streak at PSU, Borges and I went out for sushi in downtown Portland every Monday night. And when we began a winning streak at Boise State in 1994, I started having dinner at a Boise restaurant called Capers on the same night each week for several weeks.

As usual, Borges' imaginative offense was among the nation's best at the Division II level in 1991. During the regular season, we averaged 34 points and 438 yards per game. Nationally, we were ranked eighth in passing, 12th in scoring and 19th in total offense. Individually, Charles passed for 32 touchdowns and 2,619 yards and was named WFC Offensive Player of the Year and a Division II second-team All-American while running back Rodney Clemente rushed for 1,018 yards.

In our playoff opener at Civic Stadium against Northern Colorado, we jumped out to a 14-3 lead in the first quarter. But then the Bears stunned us in the second period with a pair of interceptions that were returned for touchdowns, taking a 17-14 lead at the half. Northern Colorado then widened its lead to 24-14 in the third quarter on a touchdown pass by quarterback V.J. Lechman. But Tom Mason's defense got tough and prevented any further scoring and Charles hit wide receiver Alan Boschma with a 48-yard touchdown pass in the third quarter and a 14-yard TD throw in the final period as we rallied for a 28-24 win.

Because of our continued success at the gate, we got to stay at home, as expected, for our next playoff contest—a rematch with Mankato State in the quarterfinals. In contrast to our 10-7 loss to the Mavericks at the start of the season, our playoff contest was a high-scoring affair in which we amassed 528 yards total offense. Mankato State held a 20-9 lead early in the second quarter, but Charles threw touchdown passes of 25 and 46 yards to Boschma and Henry Newson before halftime, giving us a 23-20 lead at the intermission. In the third quarter Charles threw his fourth TD pass of the game, an 11-yarder to Palomino, and running back Rais Aho, who rushed for 178 yards, added a 23-yard scoring run in the fourth period as we cruised to a 37-27 win in front of 14,275 fans. We were in the semifinals and had extended our winning streak to 10 games, which meant Sacks and I would follow our eating regimen at Viking Burger for the 10th straight week.

Throughout the 1991 season, we had a defense that bent but never broke—until our semifinal contest against eventual national champion Pittsburg State. We had a high-powered offense and 17,036 fans on our side, but it was hardly enough as the Gorillas' running attack was simply too much. The Pittsburg, Kansas, team ran roughshod over us, gaining 510 yards on the ground en route to a 53-21 thrashing. Charles completed 20 of 28 passes for 271 yards, Newson caught six passes for 149 yards and two touchdowns, and Aho rushed for more than 100 yards in his third straight playoff game, but Pittsburg State was in control from the start, vaulting to leads of 26-7 in the first quarter and 40-21 at halftime. With a devastating ground game, the aptly named Gorillas threw only nine passes and seven of their eight TDs came via the run. Pittsburg State defeated Jacksonville State 23-6 the following week for the Division II national championship.

While a shot at the national championship again eluded our team, our coaching staff had put together an impressive run with four playoff appearances in our six years at Portland State. We finished the 1991 season at 11-3 with an average home attendance of 10,144. Including our three playoff games, Charles passed for 3,527 yards and 41 touchdowns and broke seven NCAA, Western Football Conference and Portland State passing records.

WITH CHARLES AND several other key offensive players returning, "Firepower" became the slogan for our season ticket campaign in 1992. And of course I was asked to do another TV ad that spring. Wearing firefighter's gear, I appeared to be walking out of a wall of flames with a bunch of Viking football tickets smoldering in my hand. "We've got firepower!" I shouted. "Get your season tickets! They're hot!" As the earlier ads had done, this one also generated a great deal of interest among the Portland media. "It's hard to imagine [Oregon's Rich] Brooks or [Washington's Don] James looking slightly singed and wearing a fireman's suit, staggering away from a conflagration while a television camera rolls," wrote the *Oregonian's* Ken Goe. "This guy doesn't just break the mold of the grim, businesslike college football coach. He shatters it."

I suppose it's true. I don't think there are too many head coaches who have done the things I've done to promote a program. "The coach, the ringmaster, the radio personality, the commercial star, and the recruiter of both football players and the corporate dollar," was the way the *Oregonian's* Terry Frei described me in a 1992 column. "A walking public-relations agency, complete with assistants who complemented him, hoisted a beer after work with him, and likewise refused to get caught up in the paranoia of the profession."

Speaking of the coaching profession, I've often been asked if I had a role model, anyone who I considered a mentor when I was a defensive coordinator in the USFL or an assistant at the college level. No, not really. I've learned a few things from the various men I've worked for and spent time with during the early years of my career, but there is no one particular coach I've tried to emulate. Two men I highly respect are former Portland Breakers coach Dick Coury and ex-Portland State coach Mouse Davis, both of whom are assistants in the NFL. Coury is a great man, and Davis is an imaginative coach with a great football mind who has done an outstanding job throughout his career. I learned a few things about coaching from Hugh Campbell when I worked for him with the L.A. Express, and former Eastern Washington coach Dick Zornes helped me out when I was at a crossroads in my career. But no one coach really influenced me; I'd like to think I've developed my own style.

Conversely, I'm not certain if I've had a major impact on any of my longtime assistants, but I think most of them would say I have. I *do* know one thing about those guys: They're a loyal bunch. Tom Mason, Dave Stromswold and Barry Sacks have been with me all of my 11 years at Portland State and Boise State while Tom Osborne and Al Borges stayed with me for nine of those seasons. Speaking of assistant coaches, we added two to our staff in 1992. Former PSU quarterback Don Bailey, a graduate assistant the previous year, was promoted to a full-time spot to coach the receivers while Ron Gould, a former defensive back at Oregon and a grad assistant for the Ducks 1991, was hired as DB coach.

Going into the 1992 season, we considered ourselves one of the nation's top programs at the NCAA Division II level. So did a lot of the experts. We were picked No. 1 in the preseason polls published by *The Sporting News, Football Gazette* and *Football Digest* and in the top 10 in two other listings. In addition to Charles, tight end Mike Palomino and linebacker Rick Cruz were pegged as preseason All-Americans. Standout running back Rais Aho and star wide receiver Henry Newson were also returning to our talent-laden offense. Unfortunately, the 1992 season was to be the Western Football Conference's last. During that time, the NCAA had enacted new rules that prohibit a university's football and basketball programs from competing in different classifications, which meant the 11-year-old league would be forced to fold after the '92 season. PSU's plan was to compete as a Division II independent beginning in 1993.

Despite our impressive preseason credentials, we hardly looked like national title contenders through our first six games. We routed an outmanned University of Calgary club 55-0 in our season opener and beat Eastern Washington 24-21 the following week. In our win over the Eagles, however, we lost four defensive starters—linebackers Cruz and Greg Lupfer, end Tia Mavaega and free safety Ted Leach—to season-ending injuries. Then we hit a two-game skid, losing to Texas A&I 44-43 in front of 15,167 at Civic Stadium and falling to Sonoma State on the road 37-27. My counterpart in our game against the Cossacks was Tim Walsh, who replaced me as PSU's head coach two and a half months later. We downed Southern Utah 35-18 and blanked Nebraska-Kearney 44-0 in a pair of home games to improve our record to 4-2 and move to the 10th spot in the Division II national rankings. Sure, our offense was putting up plenty of points, but we were inconsistent on defense and had yet to hit our stride. But as we prepared to travel to Boise State for a non-conference game on October 24, I had a feeling that good things were going to happen.

INTERESTINGLY, OUR MATCHUP with BSU was not much more than an afterthought for the Broncos after they unexpectedly came up with an open date on their 1992 schedule when Nevada left the Big Sky Conference and decided not to play in Boise. As luck would have it, October 24 was an open date for us, and we were more than willing to fill the void in BSU's schedule.

When we reached Boise, I was struck by how much it had changed. I can still recall the scene as I walked out on the blue turf at Bronco Stadium in the late afternoon the day before our game against the Broncos. I remember gazing north over the tree-lined Boise River and a growing skyline framed by the Boise foothills. "Boy," I said wistfully, "somebody could really do some things in this place." Little did I know that in six and a half weeks, I would be Boise State's new head coach.

Prior to the 1992 season, the last time I had coached in Bronco Stadium was in 1978 as an assistant with Montana. Having coached in the West my entire career, I was quite familiar with Boise State and its reputation in the Big Sky Conference: The Broncos were the New York Yankees of the league, the football program everyone loved to hate because it had so much while the rest of the league had so little (or so it was believed). Throughout BSU's 26 years in the Big Sky, most teams got a little more cranked up to play the Broncos as opposed to other foes because they saw it as a battle between the haves and the have-nots.

When I took over as BSU's coach in 1993, I quickly discovered just how tough a place it is to coach because everybody is gunning for us every Saturday. As I work on this book, it is the fall of 1996, I'm battling cancer in Canada, and our team is in the midst of a difficult first season as a Division I-A football program in the Big West Conference. But when they played in the Big Sky from 1970 to 1995, the Broncos had it all: the best stadium, the best facilities, the best corporate backing, the most fans. When I was an assistant at Montana, we were always concerned when we faced the Broncos because we knew they almost always had superior personnel and we would have to play nearly flawless football to have any chance to win.

Despite their reputation, the Broncos were not as dominant as they once had been when we met them in '92. They were starting to struggle a little bit under head coach Skip Hall, and my perception at the time was that they hadn't done a good job of recruiting in the past few years. I thought they were starting to run short of frontline players and were not as deep as a typical Boise State football team.

I think when a really good program with a winning tradition starts having problems, it will continue to win for another season or so just because of its reputation and the fact it is used to winning. But sometimes it takes just one loss to a supposedly inferior opponent for people to suddenly realize that they don't really have that great a football team.

I think that's what happened on October 24 in Bronco Stadium.

When we came to Boise, the Broncos were ranked 16th among the nation's Division I-AA teams, riding a five-game winning streak and in the thick of the hunt for the Big Sky championship. But we thought we were going to win because we matched up extremely well against their defense, especially their secondary. Led by John Charles, we had a really outstanding offense, as good as any in Division I-AA that year. And in Al Borges we had an innovative offensive coordinator who has a real skill for exploiting an opponent's weakness. On defense we were weak against the run but pretty good against the pass, which played right into our hand because BSU had a terrible running game that year.

I remember an interview I had with Boise sportscaster Ed Vining the night before the game. He mentioned something about us being a Division II team coming in and playing Boise State and whether we thought we could "be competitive" against the Broncos. I thought that was a pretty uninformed question because I honestly thought we were the better football team. "I'm not concerned about merely being competitive tomorrow," I replied. "I think we're going to win."

Which we did the next night 51-26 as Charles shredded BSU's secondary for 444 yards passing in one of the finest performances I've ever seen by a quarterback. John completed 33 of the 40 passes he threw that night, and of the seven that weren't caught, about five of them were dropped, including one in the end zone. He was almost perfect. Our 51 points were the most ever yielded by a Boise State defense in Bronco Stadium and our 605 yards total offense was an all-time record for a BSU opponent; both records were eclipsed by Idaho four weeks later. I think one factor in our impressive performance was that we had a bye the previous week. With the extra week to prepare, Borges had time to put together several more formations, which thoroughly confused BSU's defense, and

Tom Mason was able to install twice as many stunts and blitzes on defense.

To be sure, our rout of BSU was no ordinary defeat from the Broncos' perspective. Boise State had one of the best and proudest football programs in Division I-AA with the sixth-best all-time winning percentage nationally for schools at that level before it moved to Division I-A in 1996. For a Division II club to come in and manhandle the Broncos in front of their home crowd like we did that night had to be downright embarrassing.

I have to admit, after our victory in Boise the other coaches and I talked about the possibility of going to Boise State to work because we thought Skip Hall might be in trouble. Despite our success at Portland State, we were starting to think about possibilities at other schools. It was a never-ending struggle to raise money and it was also getting tougher and tougher to find teams to play us. Idaho and Montana refused to play us anymore and with the demise of the Western Football Conference on the horizon, things were a bit unstable. Still, it was just talk among our coaching staff. Like other people, we had heard rumblings about Hall, but we didn't think his job was in serious jeopardy despite his team's loss to our club. After all, his overall performance at BSU had been relatively successful: In his five-plus years as coach, his record stood at a respectable 42-24 before the PSU game, he had never suffered a losing season, and he twice had guided the Broncos to the Division I-AA national playoffs.

Besides, we had our own concerns. We were still scrambling to get into the Division II playoffs.

OUR CHANCES OF earning a playoff berth suffered a serious setback the following week when we lost to Sacramento State 35-28 and stood at an unimpressive 5-3 after eight games. The Hornets probably weren't any better defensively than Boise State, but they had an offense that could move the ball, which hurt us because it kept our offense off the field. The next week we defeated Cal State-Northridge 35-10, but in that game Charles suffered a broken wrist and was lost for the season. Some observers thought John's injury all but ended our playoff chances, but junior Bill Matos stepped in and we never missed a beat. Matos completed 11 of 14 against Northridge in the second half and then connected on 21 of his 38 attempts for 288 yards and three TDs as we beat Cal Poly-SLO 45-31 in our final regular-season game the following week. We finished 3-1 in the WFC's final year of existence and 7-3 overall to earn a berth in the playoffs.

Charles continued PSU's proud quarterback tradition by being named the school's fifth first-team All-American at that position—joining Darren Del'Andrae, Chris Crawford, Neil Lomax and June Jones—and finishing third in the Division II Player of the Year balloting. He finished the season with 2,944 yards passing and 26 touchdowns and was also the first player to twice be named WFC Player of the Year. Our outstanding aerial game was complemented by the strong running of Rais Aho, who rushed for 1,157 yards and 21 TDs.

With playoff crowds averaging more than 14,700 since our first postseason appearance in 1987, the NCAA selection committee again awarded us the home-field advantage in our three playoff games in 1992. We always played better in the playoffs than we did during the regular season at PSU and we got it rolling again.

In our first-round contest against UC-Davis we bolted to a 28-7 lead and went on to a 42-28 victory as Aho rushed for 144 yards and two touchdowns and Matos fired four scoring passes. On that same day Idaho crushed Boise State 62-16 and Skip Hall stepped down as the Broncos' coach.

Our quarterfinals opponent was a familiar one—Texas A&I. As in the previous week, Aho rushed for 144 yards and two TDs. Both of Rais' scores were in the first half as we seized a 28-10 advantage at the intermission. Texas A&I cut our lead to 28-23 with 13 points in the third quarter, but Matos and Henry Newson combined on a 20-yard touchdown pass in the final period for a 35-23 lead. The Javelinas scored late in the game, but it wasn't enough as we won 35-30 in front of 12,657 fans. Like we had done in 1988, we avenged a regular-season loss to the Javelinas with a playoff victory. And similar to the '88 playoff game against Texas A&I, we jumped out to a big lead and held on for the win. Our victory set up a rematch at home with defending national champ Pittsburg State, which had thrashed us in the previous year's semis.

In what turned out to be our coaching staff's final game at Portland State, we suffered one of the toughest losses I can remember. With a crowd of 13,180 looking on, we entered the fourth quarter with a 38-26 lead after Matos hit Mike Palomino with an 18-yard touchdown late in the third period. We were 15 minutes away from a return trip to Florence, Alabama, and the Division II title game. But it wasn't to be. The Gorillas' Ronald Moore, who had run wild against our defense the entire game, scored on a two-yard run to cut our lead to 38-33. He then stunned the entire stadium with a 93-yard dash late in the game to lift his team to a 41-38 triumph. Moore rushed for an astounding 379 yards and five touchdowns as the Gorillas denied us a shot at the national championship for the second consecutive year. Led by Aho's 145 yards on the ground and Matos' 331 yards in the air our offense piled up 499 total yards and certainly played well enough to win. But we blew it with some bad defense and costly penalties. As I mentioned, our run defense had been our Achilles' heel ever since we lost four starters early in the season, and it finally caught up with us as the Gorillas rushed for 558 yards and threw the ball only four times. With the win, Pittsburg State advanced to a rematch in the championship game with Jacksonville State. Only this time the Gamecocks took the title with a 17-13 triumph the following week.

We finished 9-4 in 1992 and reached the Division II playoffs five of our seven years at Portland State. With an average of 12,371 fans per game, the '92 season also marked the fourth time that we set a regular-season attendance record. When all was said and done, our staff left Portland State having won 70 percent of our games with an impressive 63-26-2 record—the fifth-best in Division II history. We won five Western Football Conference titles and I collected seven coach of the year awards.

Our semifinal setback to Pittsburg State was devastating, to say the least. But I've always tried not to dwell too long on defeats, even tough ones like that. Besides, I quickly had to turn my full attention to another matter: The head coaching job at Boise State.

Chapter 11

Bound for Boise

I watched the coaching situation at Boise State with growing interest after we defeated the Broncos in late October. Skip Hall's critics had become more vocal. It wasn't enough that he was an unforgivable 0-5 against archrival Idaho, they griped, now he was losing to *Division II* teams. The criticism escalated as the Broncos' tailspin continued with losses to Big Sky opponents Montana State and Eastern Washington.

I had heard enough rumors and knew enough about the impatience of Boise State football fans to figure Hall was in trouble as the Idaho-BSU game approached. When the Broncos finished 5-6 in 1986, their first losing season in 40 years, fourth-year coach Lyle Setencich was sent packing despite the fact he had posted winning records the previous three years. Many presumed the same fate awaited Hall if he didn't figure out a way to defeat the Vandals on November 21. Assuming Hall's days were numbered, I decided to send my résumé to BSU athletic director Gene Bleymaier.

The Vandals showed no mercy; their 62-16 annihilation of Boise State was the worst defeat in school history. BSU's 1992 campaign ended with a four-game losing streak and a 5-6 record, the school's second losing season since 1946. The drubbing in Bronco Stadium also marked Idaho's 11th consecutive win over Boise State, dropping Hall's record against the Vandals to 0-6. To the surprise of no one, Hall resigned "under pressure" a few hours after the game.

On the same day that Hall was stepping down, I was leading Portland State to a first-round victory over UC-Davis in the Division II playoffs—a fact I hoped wasn't lost on those who would have to find a replacement for Hall. It certainly wasn't lost on the media. "Hall Resigns," announced the headline on the front page of the *Idaho Statesman*, Boise's daily newspaper, the morning after BSU's loss to UI. In the same day's sports section was another headline: "Two Possible Successors: Pokey Allen, Gregg Smith."

Speculation was also running high in Portland. Two days after BSU's loss to Idaho, *Oregonian* columnist Terry Frei wrote the following: "Portland State's Pokey Allen helped force the Saturday resignation of Boise State's Skip Hall, so don't be shocked if Allen becomes a bona fide candidate for the job at the Big Sky Conference school. When PSU manhandled Division I-AA Boise State 51-26 on the road last month, it heated up the previously scattered grumblings about Hall, whose Broncos dropped to 5-3 at the time and would [not win again that season].

"The performance of the Vikings also impressed a lot of folks in Boise, who openly wondered how a bus-riding, Division II program could come in and so decisively beat perhaps the most well-heeled I-AA operation in the nation. The PSU coaches were openly envious of the Broncos' facilities and resources in the biggest market in the Big Sky. If Allen decides that he can't land a decent Division I-A head coaching job, and decides he isn't anchored in Portland with the Vikings or a possible Canadian Football League franchise, then Boise State makes sense. For both sides."

Frei was on to something, but I wasn't about to say anything. As much as I dislike secrecy, I felt I had to be somewhat vague about my interest in the Boise State position. I wasn't trying to play games, but with our team in the Division II playoffs, my assistant coaches and I feared that any publicity about my candidacy for another job would be a huge distraction to our players as we geared up for another run at the national championship. In his column, Frei reported that I hadn't spoken with anyone connected with the BSU program, which at the time was true. "I know my name's being mentioned," I said to Frei. "But then my name's mentioned for every job." A week later, however, I was definitely in the running—even though we were still trying to keep my dealings with BSU under wraps.

Within a week and a half of the UI-BSU game, the number of candidates had been narrowed to five. According to the media, the list consisted of New Mexico State head coach Jim Hess, Missouri offensive coordinator Dirk Koetter, BSU assistant athletic director Herb Criner, University of Miami assistant head coach Gregg Smith and me. Both Koetter and Smith had strong Idaho ties. Both played high school and college football in the state (Koetter at Highland of Pocatello and Idaho State; Smith at Moscow High and UI) and both served as head high school coaches in Idaho before advancing to the college ranks. Initially, I didn't think I had much of a chance because some big-money boosters—led by billionaire J.R. Simplot and prominent Boise businessmen Allen Noble and Jon Miller— wanted Smith. In fact, in the December 2 issue of the *Idaho Statesman*, sports editor John Millman reported that a group of boosters had flown from Boise to San Diego—where Miami had played San Diego State the previous weekend—in Simplot's private plane, presumably to court Smith.

That same weekend Portland State defeated Texas A&I in the Division II quarterfinals; a day or so later I surreptitiously flew into Boise to interview for the BSU job. Actually, I think my first "interview" took place October 24 with Portland State's win over Boise State. When a Division II team comes into Bronco Stadium and moves the football at will against a BSU defense, people sit up and take notice. Would I have been a candidate for Skip Hall's vacated position had we not embarrassed his team a month earlier? No question about it, I never would have had a chance.

I was in Boise for only a day because I had to get back to my team to prepare for our semifinal contest against Pittsburg State. During my visit I met with the 22-person search committee that was named by Larry Selland, then BSU's acting president. Chaired by Bleymaier, there were some really good people on the committee, men like Boise businessman Jim Nelson, former BSU football coach and athletic director Lyle Smith, team physician George Wade and Steve Vogel, a former BSU player and head coach at Capital High School in Boise.

During my brief visit to Boise and in the ensuing days in Portland, I heard rumors that Smith and I were the front-runners. But I couldn't give it too much thought because I was still trying to coach Portland State to the Division II national championship. Within a day or so of my visit, my candidacy for the Boise State job had become widely known—and speculation was running rampant. Of particular interest to the *Statesman's* Millman was the power and influence of the men who wanted Smith.

"Allen charmed the search committee," wrote Millman in his December 2 column, "but the ultimate decision is Bleymaier's. Will Bleymaier snub the big-money boosters and pick Pokey? It's not like he's settling for leftovers. Or will Bleymaier take Smith, the top assistant from the top college football program in the country? ... Guaranteed, when Bleymaier makes his announcement ... somebody's not going to like it.

"Big money won't like the selection of Allen, and big money talks ... Anti-big money will resent the selection of Smith, and there's power in the people. It's Bleymaier's call, and it's a tough one. No doubt he'll do what he believes is best for the program and the community. It's crucial he makes it clear the choice was his with the blessing of the search committee. No doubt he will, even if his choice is Gregg Smith."

Selland and Bleymaier were in quite a dilemma. I think they were under some real pressure because of the clout wielded by those who wanted Smith as the Broncos' next coach. I knew Selland and Bleymaier wanted to hire somebody by the second week of December, and I definitely wanted a shot at the job.

But there was still that little matter of PSU's appearance in the Division II semifinals on December 5. I'm not sure what would have happened had we won that game against Pittsburg State, but it became academic when the Gorillas rallied to beat us 41-38. You know, sometimes I think I might have been too distracted trying to get the BSU job. Maybe if I had given the task at hand my undivided attention we might have beaten Pittsburg State and made another trip to Florence, Alabama, and won that elusive national championship.

With our season over at PSU, I flew back to Boise on Tuesday, December 8, for a second interview. It was apparent the choice was down to Smith and me.

I'm not sure if most people realize what a big deal the head coaching job at Boise State is. When BSU played in Division I-AA, it was among the most coveted head coaching jobs in the nation at that level. I can't say for sure, but I don't think Gregg Smith would have applied for too many I-AA head coaching positions. I mean, he was the assistant head coach at Miami, which happened to be the top-ranked team in the nation at the time. I don't think he would have applied for the head job at Montana or even Idaho, his alma mater, for that matter. But Boise State was—and still is—a completely different deal. The job has everything. Boise is a great place to live and BSU is a great place to coach with incredible community support and outstanding facilities and resources— the whole package. As I've said before, BSU is having a tough time in 1996, its first year at the Division I-A level, but there's no question in my mind that the Broncos will eventually be as competitive in Division I-A as they were in I-AA. The program just has too many positives for it not to excel.

Anyway, when I returned to Boise I had dinner with Jon Miller, Allen Noble and J.R. Simplot. Like I said, Miller and Noble, both of whom became friends of mine, are among the more affluent members of the Boise business community. And calling Simplot a "wealthy" businessman is like calling Michael Jordan a "pretty good" basketball player. Now in his late 80s, Simplot created and developed an agriculture-based business empire that has made him one of the richest men in the world. Even though Simplot, Noble and Miller weren't on BSU's search committee, it was obvious they carried a certain amount of influence in the selection process. I came to that conclusion because it was Bleymaier who chauffeured me to Miller's home for my dinner engagement that evening. My get-together with the three boosters was enjoyable and I think I said all the right things, but I still didn't think I was going to get the job.

On the morning of December 9 I met with a few more people at Boise State and then took a ride through Boise to look at houses with assistant athletic director Dave Jerome. I wasn't really interested in house hunting because I was still pretty pessimistic about my chances, but I figured I'd better go. Jerome and I got back to the Varsity Center around noon and Bleymaier called me into his office. "The job's yours if you want it," he said. I guess he caught me a little off guard because right up until that moment, I really thought Smith was going to be the choice. "Yeah, I want it," I said.

I don't know if Simplot, Noble and Miller changed their minds after our dinner meeting or if Bleymaier went with me against their wishes. I think in a way maybe their favoritism toward Smith worked to my advantage. I'm just guessing here, but I think maybe Gene didn't want to be dictated to by some big-money boosters. I don't know what politics were involved in the decision, but I've always had a feeling that something happened in the final hours before I was hired because BSU wrestling coach Mike Young, who would become one of my best friends in Boise, later told me he heard that someone from Boise called Smith that morning and said, "Congratulations, you got the job." Again, I'm just guessing, but I think there were some last-minute, behind-the-scenes dealings that took place which worked in my favor; I'm not sure what. I really have never talked to Gene at length about why he picked me over Smith; I was just happy he did. Things worked out for Smith. He remained with Miami head coach Dennis Erickson and is now an assistant coach under Erickson with the NFL's Seattle Seahawks.

I assume I had three factors working in my favor: my head coaching experience, which Smith didn't have; the fact our staff had won more than 70 percent of our games at PSU; and our impressive win over Boise State earlier that season. I suppose my personality helped, too. I think Boise State was looking for a different style than that of the straight-laced Skip Hall, and perhaps my reputation as a fun-loving type who could party hard, win football games and have a lot of fun in the process worked to my benefit. That certainly appeared to be the impression I gave Eldon Edmundson, former dean of BSU's College of Health Science and a member of the selection committee. When he talked to a writer about the interview process, Edmundson said, "In my opinion, the finalists for the job seemed to be pretty equal as far as X's and O's. Pokey seemed to be an excellent tactical coach, but what he also brought to the table was the ability to come across as a coach who could make football fun—for the fans, the coaches, the players, the community. Pokey told the committee, 'Hey, we won't win every game, but I guarantee we'll have fun trying.' I can't speak for the entire committee, but I think that impressed a lot of people."

My base salary was $69,000, only $1,000 more than what I was making at Portland State, but I didn't care. In fact, when the *Oregonian* asked me how much I would be making at Boise State, I said, "I don't know. He [Bleymaier] offered me the job, and I took it."

I think Bleymaier might have been aware of my reputation as a flake—perhaps he had heard the story of my short-lived coaching stint at Weber State in 1980—because what followed was kind of amusing. Right after Gene and I shook hands on the deal, I suddenly remembered that I had promised one of our big boosters in Portland that I would call him right away to let him know about my decision. "Gene," I said to Bleymaier, "before we alert the media I have to call this guy." All of a sudden Bleymaier got this real concerned look on his face. "You're not backing out now, are you?" he asked. "No," I assured him, "I'm your coach. I just need to make a phone call first."

That afternoon, the university announced my hiring at a press conference in the BSU Student Union. As much as I enjoyed the many zany promotions we concocted to generate fan interest at Portland State, I was thrilled to be with a program that didn't require such marketing efforts. Now, I was with a program where the school's 23,000-seat stadium was at or near capacity for almost every game.

"I'm in utopia," I said to the reporters and boosters who had gathered for the announcement. "I'm someplace where people care about football. I'm excited about being here. At Portland State I spent five years getting people to care. Not whether we won, just to care. You don't have that problem here. I could have applied for a lot of jobs and I didn't. I want this job. I want to be at Boise State and coach for the Broncos. I think Boise State is one of the premier jobs. If you're a coach and you don't look at Boise State as [an attractive] job, you're crazy."

Speaking of crazy, things got a little strange for a day or two when I returned to Portland. But then, our coaching staff was known for its strangeness, so why should our final days at PSU have been any different? I told the Boise media that I expected most of my assistants to follow me to Boise. I was hoping offensive coordinator Al Borges would come, too. But I knew Portland State considered him the primary candidate to replace me as the school's head coach. "Al Borges has proven he's a great offensive coach. ... He does a great job. I think he should be selected for the PSU job," I told the *Oregonian* when I returned to Portland on Thursday, December 10. "But I won't kid you. I'm trying to get him to go to Boise."

The *Oregonian's* Terry Frei also thought Al should be the Vikings' top choice. "[PSU's] first priority should be an all-out blitz on Borges," Frei wrote. "Borges ran the entertaining offense, he shook many of the same hands as Allen, he has instant credibility in the community, and he probably would be a great head coach."

That same afternoon I met individually with my assistant coaches and said I wanted each of them to make a commitment, one way or the other, by noon Friday. That night, a group of friends threw a going-away party for me and the other coaches at Jake's in Portland. During the course of the evening Borges came up to me and said, "Would you mind if I went after the Portland State job?" I said, "Al, I want what's best for you. If that's what you want, and you don't want to join us in Boise, I understand perfectly. I'll even back you for the Portland State job if that's your decision." I was still hoping, however, that Al would join me at BSU.

I went home that night not thinking much about my conversation with Al. But the next morning I got a real shock. Barb and I were driving to work; she was behind the wheel and I was casually reading the paper until I came to the *Oregonian's* sports section. The headline of the lead story read, "Borges to accept PSU job." The article, written by Ken Goe, reported that Al had accepted Portland State athletic director Randy Nordlof's job offer late Thursday night—apparently after our conversation at Jake's— and that a formal announcement would be made that afternoon. "Borges was initially reluctant to be considered for PSU's head job," Goe wrote. "By Thursday afternoon he seemed to be warming to the idea."

I told Barb to pull over, and I hopped out and called Bleymaier from a pay phone. "We've lost our offensive coordinator," I told Gene. Borges wasn't part of my agreement with BSU, but I knew many people in Boise were excited about having him on the Bronco staff, so I thought it best to tell Bleymaier the news right away. When I arrived at the football offices at Portland State a few minutes later there was all kinds of commotion because Al was trying to put a staff together that included some of the coaches I had planned to bring to Boise.

The first thing I did was call defensive coordinator Tom Mason into my office. "This might turn a little ugly," I said to Tom. "I want to take you guys to Boise and I suppose Al wants to keep some of you here. I'm not sure what's going to happen." Mason looked at me and said, "No problem, I'm going with you." So after Al talked to some of the coaches, I called them into my office to see what kind of staff I was going to have at Boise State. I even called a coach whom I thought could replace Borges as my offensive coordinator. I figured Mason and Dave Stromswold would come with me, but I wasn't sure about the others. And they only had until noon to make up their minds.

But around 10:30 a.m. Borges walked into my office. He said he had just informed Nordlof that he had rescinded his acceptance of the PSU job and wanted to remain my offensive coordinator. The people at Portland State have always been a class act, and they took Al's decision in stride.

"Al called me late last night and told me he would take the job," Nordlof told the *Oregonian* later that day. "This morning when he got here he said he had tossed and turned all night and just wasn't comfortable with the situation."

"There were no outside influences that entered into this," Borges said in the same article, published on Saturday, December 12. "Pokey has been awesome all the way through it. Randy has been awesome all the way through it. It wasn't so much that I didn't think I could do it. It was more that I didn't want to do it. ... The decision I'm making now is a little self-ish. I'm doing what I think is right for me. The thing I feel the worst about is that I know I led some people on. But I'm glad I'm doing this because it would have been unfair to myself and, more importantly, unfair to the players. To do this job right your heart has to be in it. I'm not sure mine was and that would have been reflected in what happened on the field."

So within two and a half hours, I went from losing my offensive co-ordinator, to trying to find a new one, to having Al back on our staff. Sheepishly, I called Bleymaier again. "Hey, Gene," I said. "It's Pokey. Heh-heh. Uh ... remember that phone call I made earlier this morning? Heh-heh. Um ... guess what? Al changed his mind. He's er ... coming with us to Boise State after all. Great, huh?" I imagined poor Gene at the other end of the line, shaking his head and wondering what kind of nitwit he had hired.

I don't mean to brag, but I think part of Borges' decision was the realization that he had a tough act to follow at PSU. I'm not saying I'm the greatest football coach who ever blew a whistle, but I had developed quite a following in Portland, and even *I* wouldn't have wanted to replace me at Portland State. Al also knew that working for a Division I-AA program allowed him, and the rest of our staff for that matter, to step out from the

Division II shadows. I look at it this way: Borges had to go to a Division I-AA school before he could get a Division I-A job. Once we became Division I-AA coaches, we were no longer outcasts in the eyes of Division I-A schools. I think Al Borges has one of the most imaginative offensive minds in football, and he wasn't any different a coach at Portland State than he was at Boise State. But all of a sudden he was good enough to get the offensive coordinator's job at Oregon in 1995 and at UCLA in '96. Before that, nobody would hire him at the I-A level even though his offensive teams were always statistically ranked near the top nationally in Division II for passing yards, total offense and scoring. I mean, perception is everything.

With Borges back on board, our coaching staff was intact for our move to BSU. A few days later the seven of us—Borges, Tom Mason, Dave Stromswold, Barry Sacks, Ron Gould, Tom Osborne and me—loaded up a van and headed off to our new lives in Boise. We were later joined by two restricted-earnings coaches—Don Bailey, who played quarterback and coached for me at Portland State, and Pete Kwiatkowski, an All-American defensive tackle for BSU in 1987 and the lone holdover from Skip Hall's staff. Coming into a new program, we were behind schedule in regard to recruiting. We were working off our recruitment list from Portland State, but now we were up a level and trying to re-evaluate the players we were going after to determine if they could play I-AA football.

IN APRIL 1993, early in our inaugural spring drills at Boise State, I quickly concluded that Skip Hall and his assistants didn't lose because they couldn't coach; it was because they didn't recruit well during their last two or three seasons. It wasn't that Hall and his staff didn't have *any* blue-chip players, they just didn't have enough of them.

"Jeez," I said during a spring coaches' meeting, "I wished I had looked at the films a little better before I took this position; I didn't realize we were going to have a total rebuilding job ahead of us." I just assumed the BSU football program, with its outstanding facilities and winning tradition, would have plenty of good, young players waiting in the wings. Boy, was I wrong. Oh sure, there was a handful of key performers coming back from Hall's 1992 squad—wide receivers Mike Wilson and Jarett Hausske, defensive tackles Chris Shepherd and Kimo von Oelhoffen, defensive backs DaWuan Miller and Rashid Gayle, linebacker Brian Smith and a few others—but our overall lack of talent and depth was alarming.

To fill some of the holes in our lineup we signed a handful of junior college imports—linebacker Stefan Reid, safety Chris Cook, running back

Willie Bowens and quarterback Lee Schrack—along with transfers Joe O'Brien, a defensive end from Santa Clara, and Cliff Robinson, a linebacker from Washington State. But I still didn't think we had anywhere near the number of quality players we needed to be competitive. To make matters worse, senior Travis Stuart, BSU's starting quarterback in 1992, left the team. At the conclusion of our spring practices, some members of our staff still thought we could win a fair share of our games that fall; I wasn't as optimistic. Truth be told, I had a strong feeling our first year at Boise State was going to be a long one.

And long it was. On September 4, 1993, we defeated Rhode Island 31-10 in my first game as BSU's head coach. But from there it was all down-hill. We got routed by Nevada 38-10 the following week before returning home to down Northeastern 27-13 as Bowens rushed for 211 yards. After a 30-7 loss to Stephen F. Austin at home on September 25 we stood at 2-2. In our next game, a road contest at Montana, Al Borges and I decided to start freshmen Tony Hilde and Ryan Ikebe at quarterback and wide receiver, respectively. We had hoped to redshirt both Tony and Ryan that year, but they were pressed into service because of injuries and lack of depth on offense. Although we got routed by the Grizzlies 38-24, Hilde was outstanding, completing 21 of 38 passes for 388 yards and a 45-yard touchdown pass to Ikebe. After their impressive debuts, Hilde and Ikebe stayed in the starting lineup—and over the next three and a half seasons they would go on to become one of the best QB-wideout combinations in BSU history.

But the defeats continued to mount. The following week we lost 23-9 to Northern Arizona at home, which marked the first time I had ever lost three straight games as a head coach, then Weber State edged us 21-14 with a game-winning touchdown in the final seconds. At least one good thing happened in the middle of that dreadful season: Barbara gave birth to our daughter, Taylor Elizabeth, on Sunday, October 17. I was a dad at age 50.

As the losses piled up that year I definitely needed all the so-called charm and humor I could muster to keep the critics at bay. I suppose my "engaging personality," as the media called it, helped stave off some of the criticism, but I knew it was only a matter of time before the honey-moon would be over if things didn't improve—fast.

"This is not a place where you can take a lot of time to get it going," I told the *Oregonian's* Steve Brandon the week after our loss to Weber State. "They want a winner, and they're used to having good offenses. We'd better be good by next year." As a whole, BSU fans are an unforgiving bunch;

most of them, however, seemed to like me and were willing to give our staff the benefit of the doubt that season. "Support for the new Allen regime has been strong so far," Brandon wrote. "Allen is not as revered as he was in Portland, but he is popular. People see him as genuine."

I knew we were going to be bad in 1993, but not *that* bad. We were lousy on offense but had some decent talent on defense; the problem was we didn't play hard all the time. By midseason only six of the 14 returning first stringers from the '92 squad were still starting and six true freshmen had seen action. In retrospect, I think we could have won a few more games that year, but we didn't get any breaks, and it always seems like the teams that need the breaks never get them. But I don't mean to make excuses; any way you look at it, we were awful in 1993. It was embarrassing and frustrating, and I knew we would have to take drastic measures to make sure our nightmare didn't repeat itself in 1994. Sometime late in the season I remember saying to Tom Mason and Al Borges, "Hey, we can't do what we originally planned to do and bring in 10 junior college transfers and 15 freshmen and straighten it out for next year. We won't survive doing it that way. We have to bring in *lots* of JC players and get rid of a lot of people for next season. Otherwise, I don't think we'll be here two years from now."

Six days after Taylor was born we beat Idaho State 34-27, but our misery continued as we lost to Montana State 42-21 and Eastern Washington 28-17. Played in front of a sparse crowd of 10,238, the lowest turnout in Bronco Stadium in 20 years, our November 13 loss to Dick Zornes' Eagles was the lowest point in a season full of low points. By that time, the pressure had become palpable. "Teams do not have to beat us, we beat ourselves. I feel incredibly bad for the city of Boise," I told Phil Smith of the *Idaho Statesman* after the game. Then, like I've been known to do, I blurted out what was really on my mind: "Give me one more year and I'll straighten it out or I'll be gone. I can't take a year like this again. If we don't straighten it out next year, you won't have to worry about [long-term] contracts or anything else." Pretty strong words, but I wasn't kidding. I've never believed in a long rebuilding program. A week later the 1993 season mercifully ended as we lost to Idaho 49-16. It was the Vandals' 12th consecutive win over Boise State.

THE '93 SEASON had been a disaster on the football field and my personal life wasn't much better. Despite the birth of our daughter, Barb and I weren't getting along; the pressure to win that year grew so intense it began to take an enormous toll on our marriage. Coaching is a tough business to begin with; it will test even the best of marriages. The work is demanding, time-consuming and full of pressure. Coaches and their spouses have to have the right attitude to make their marriage work, and I guess we didn't have it.

Like most relationships, ours was great at first. When Barb and I first started dating, I quickly realized that she had—and still has—a lot of qualities that I had never previously looked for in a woman. With her good looks, poise and business acumen, she has a presence about her that really impresses people. Because of our age difference, I think some people initially assumed, "Oh, there's Pokey taking out another young one again." But Barb was different, and it was never more apparent than one evening early in our courtship when I took her to a banquet hosted by Portland State's central administration. The place was full of important company executives and other VIPs. As I took her around and introduced her to people, it became quite evident that she was in her element. I mean, here was this young, attractive, up-and-coming businesswoman who could talk to these corporate bigwigs and high-powered types, some more than twice her age, in their own lingo like she was one of them. It suddenly dawned on me: She *was* one of them.

Barb is a tremendous person, and our courtship and the first two years of marriage were lots of fun. We ran together. We had parties on the houseboat. It was a great life in Portland. But to be perfectly honest, deep down inside, I don't think I ever wanted to get married. Barb was different than any other woman I had had a relationship with; I thought that if I were going to get married again, she would be the one. But after we had been married for a few years, it was like … well, *being married*.

I think Barb assumed I would become more like a normal husband after awhile. But I don't think I'm ever going to be like that. I just don't think I'm cut out for marriage. I'm not sure what qualities you need to be a good husband, but I don't think I have any of them. In retrospect, marriage has always struck me as very boring. I still feel that way. Most marriages I see are boring. I also have this philosophy: The qualities many women liked in their husbands before they were married are the same characteristics they dislike after the wedding. When a couple is dating it's OK for the guy to dance and party and to be funny and outgoing and charming. But after they get married, a lot of women say, "Do you have to be so damn charming and have so much fun?"

And one thing I'm not is a recluse. I love being around people. I thoroughly enjoyed having barbecues on the houseboat with 15 to 20 people where everybody brought a dish. And if people didn't come to our home,

I would go to them, a habit I think Barb grew tired of. But, hey, I enjoy talking to people and being in bars. I enjoy the camaraderie. I rarely over-indulge and I've never been out of control, but I have always enjoyed that atmosphere. It's not like I was out all night or out carousing, but I admit I *was* gone a lot. Meeting lots of people in local establishments helped our football program at Portland State and made me successful as a coach; I really didn't feel I needed to stop. I guess the bottom line was this: Barb wanted me to change and I wasn't willing to do so.

So when we moved to Boise in 1993 we were already having prob-lems. And the situation was exacerbated when we started losing football games left and right. We lived in a fishbowl in Boise—where losing foot-ball games is akin to high treason—and the pressure to win grew intense. It was a terrible time for me, and a terrible time for Barbara to be around me. In a town where the university's head football coach is the most pub-lic of figures, our life was full of tension and stress. The following spring Barb and I separated for a week or two because things were going so poorly, but it didn't help much. You know, being a football coach's wife is not good even in the best of times, and being *my* wife is really not good even in the best of times.

Finally, in the late summer of 1994 Barbara and I thought it best if we separated; Barb took Taylor and moved to Missoula where she could be with family and run her business as a commercial lender for a finance company. Once we had made the decision not to live together Barb wanted to leave town. And I certainly understood; being Pokey Allen's estranged wife would not be easy in Boise. She also thought I was being unfaithful, which wasn't the case at the time. However, I did have an affair in Boise several months earlier. Even so, our split was amicable, and our relation-ship now is quite good. We saw each other quite a bit after the move be-cause she was coming down to Boise on business.

I did some things I shouldn't have while I was married, but let me dispel a few rumors here: There was gossip that Barbara caught me with someone else while she was pregnant with Taylor. That never happened. There was also a rumor going around that I had been sleeping with a booster's wife. I have never been with a booster's wife or anybody else's wife. I mean, this was the kind of groundless and unjustified crap Barb and I had to put up with; I don't blame her for wanting to leave Boise once we decided to split up.

Looking back, I think we had different priorities that we should have discussed before we got married. First, she wanted to have a lot of chil-dren, and I knew I wasn't going to have more than one.

But I love the one I have. I'm biased, but I think Taylor is precious. I'm just sick that I can't see more of her.

She's about to turn three as I work on this book in Vancouver in October of 1996. I try to call her at her daycare in Missoula every day on my cellular phone during my daily drive to radiation treatment. Right now she can sing nine songs, and the other day she wanted to sing all nine to me. This past summer I picked her up in Missoula two or three times and drove her up to the cabin on Flathead Lake.

I sometimes get teary-eyed when I'm talking to Taylor or when I talk to Barbara about her. I know I wasn't a very good husband to Taylor's mom, but I think I'm going to be a great father. I care and I want to be around her and I want to talk to her about things while she's growing up. I think being a dad has improved me as a person. And I like being a parent more than I thought I would. I mean, I like having a little daughter who loves me unconditionally. Being Taylor's dad makes me want to live. I want to be there when she graduates from high school and college and when she gets married. I hope I can live 20 more years to see those things, but right now I'm not sure.

Chapter 12

A Magical Season

BSU football is serious business in Boise. The Broncos have a storied tradition and a rich history of success that includes the Division I-AA national championship in 1980. If our coaching staff would have attempted to produce a winner at Boise State the long-term way, which most programs do by primarily recruiting and signing first-year players, we would have needed five-year contracts to protect our jobs. But after our disastrous first year, I didn't think we had that kind of time. Like I told Al Borges and Tom Mason near the end of the 1993 season, we weren't going to be at BSU very long if we didn't straighten things out in a hurry.

I said as much following the 1993 Eastern Washington game and again in an article written by then *Idaho Statesman* sports editor Art Lawler in the summer of 1994. "It may be more in his mind than anywhere else," Lawler wrote, "but the BSU football coach feels he's got a year to rebuild his team. ... Most people think the pressure by Allen is largely self-inflicted, but [a booster] adds, 'If he doesn't win this year, I think he'll be out of here. But that's just something Pokey has put on himself. Most people I know realize a coach needs at least three years to build his program.'" The pressure was incredible. We had been with the program for one season, and already there were grumblings. As Lawler surmised, much of it I brought on myself—"I think we'll need to be 6-5 or 7-4 this year, and be real competitive; I don't think we can be below .500 and cut it," I said in his article—but I also know that BSU football fans are not a patient lot, and I simply didn't believe we would be given the kind of time necessary to build through freshman class after freshman class.

So right after the '93 season I sent Barry Sacks out on the junior college recruiting trail in search of new talent to fill our immediate needs. Another early and unpleasant task was to get rid of some of the returning players whom the other coaches and I decided did not fit into our plans. How did we "convince" them to leave the program? I called each one in and told him that we didn't think he could play here anymore, that we weren't going to renew his scholarship, or that his scholarship was being cut from full to half. (NCAA regulations allow student-athletes who lose their scholarships to appeal such decisions, but they rarely do and usually end up leaving.) We had to do the same thing at Portland State after our first year. It's not an enjoyable chore, but schools at the Division I-AA and II levels simply don't have enough scholarships to be charitable. If you have people on your roster who you don't think can play, it's only fair to the players and the program to act accordingly. That's what we did.

Meanwhile, Sacks started lining up junior college prospects in an effort to shore up some of our team's weaknesses. Sacks is one of the best recruiters I have ever been around; by dint of personality and salesmanship he helped bring in a bunch of talented athletes to take a look at BSU's campus, view the athletic department's facilities and meet our coaches and players.

Despite our team's abysmal performance in 1993, we had a pretty good nucleus of talented and tough kids coming back for the '94 campaign: quarterback Tony Hilde; wide receivers Lee Schrack (whom we converted from quarterback), Ryan Ikebe and Jarett Hausske; DBs DaWuan Miller, Chris Cook and Rashid Gayle; defensive linemen Sione Fifita, Chris Shepherd and Joe O'Brien; kicker Greg Erickson; and linebackers Stefan Reid and Brian Smith. An added dimension was the senior leadership provided by Cook, Hausske, Schrack, Reid and O'Brien—a characteristic that was missing from our team the previous year. Any college sports program's best salesmen are the players. And those seniors, along with Smith, a junior, took it upon themselves to help us successfully recruit many of the JC players who joined us for the 1994 season. I found it especially gratifying to learn that guys such as Smith, Miller, Gayle, Erickson and Hausske— guys who initially came to BSU to play for Skip Hall—were among our program's most vocal advocates.

They must have said the right things because we had an outstanding recruiting season, signing 21 junior college transfers. As things turned out, most of our JC guys were key performers on our 1994 team, which is rare indeed. Usually, schools will recruit 12 or so junior college players and hope that maybe six will have an impact on their program the following two years. But in 1994, about 16 former JC players helped us to the national championship game. Another key addition to our program was strength coach Joe Kenn, who brought a new mind-set to the team's off-season conditioning program. Joe's serious approach to weight training— his motto is you either change the attitude or change the people—was a major factor in our success in 1994. After assessing our personnel during the first few days of spring drills in April, there was no question that we were going to be a much improved team.

When our twice-a-day summer drills rolled around in August, our coaching staff decided to hold our second practice of each day in the evenings, which really seemed to help. By escaping the broiling midday sun, the practices didn't seem as arduous as they had been the previous year when we went mornings and afternoons. We just seemed to push the right buttons that year. You know, the 1994 team was one of the most interesting groups I have ever coached. It was a great bunch of players with some real leaders showing the way by word and example. Like I said, I think the word "magic" is tossed around way too much, but during our double days that summer, we had a couple of sessions where I could tell something special was happening. We cared. We worked hard. We were a team in the real sense of the word. Morale was high among the players and coaches, and it was contagious. I remember one morning during double sessions, standing in the middle of practice observing the spirit and enthusiasm all around me. "Hey, gang," I shouted to the entire team, "we have a shot!" I didn't say a shot at what … because I wasn't sure myself.

But by the time the season was ready to start on September 3, I felt we were going to be a pretty good football team. Not great by any means, but I thought something like a 7-4 record and a second- or third-place finish in the Big Sky and an outside shot at the Division I-AA playoffs was not out of the question. I even thought we had a good chance to beat Idaho.

IN OUR SEASON opener against Northeastern we trailed 26-21 in the third quarter before rallying to win 36-26. K.C. Adams—a junior running back who was academically ineligible the previous season—rushed for 172 yards, and Chris Shepherd blocked a 28-yard field goal attempt that would have tied the game at 29 in the fourth quarter before Adams sealed the victory with his third touchdown of the game. In our second game against Cal State-Northridge we were tied at 19 early in the fourth quarter before we broke the game open with a pair of huge scoring plays less than two minutes apart—an 84-yard pass from Tony Hilde to Jarett Hausske and Adams' 79-yard punt return. Adams scored twice, rushed for 129 yards and returned three punts for 101 yards in our 40-19 victory over the Matadors.

As the 1994 season was unfolding, Boise State was in the final stages of a prolonged effort to attain I-A status in football. In mid-September the university was officially extended an invitation to join the Division I-A

Big West Conference, a move that in two years would place us in the upper echelon of college football.

Ironically, a few days before BSU accepted the Big West's offer, our team was scheduled to meet former Big Sky and future Big West foe Nevada. Before the season started the other coaches and I knew our matchup with the Wolf Pack would be one of our biggest challenges because coach Chris Ault had put together another excellent team—probably better than the squad that beat us by four touchdowns in Reno the previous year. After nearly three decades of coaching, I think I have developed an ability to gauge my team's mental preparedness for an important game. And despite our concerns about the talent-laden Wolf Pack, I liked what I saw as we got ready for our September 17 showdown with Nevada in Bronco Stadium. I think many college football games are won by what takes place on the practice field on Monday through Thursday—not on Friday or the Saturday morning of game day. And by the end of our practice on Thursday, September 15, I knew we were going to have a good game against Nevada—although I still had serious doubts if we had enough firepower to actually win.

Coaching can be a nasty business at times, but games like the one we played that night against Nevada make it all worthwhile. I love big games against formidable opponents, and I think preparing a team for an important matchup is one of the greatest challenges a coach can face. I thoroughly enjoy the strategic aspects of the coaching profession; it's the day-to-day duties—the discipline, the paperwork, the travel—that can wear you down at times. To be sure, you don't get the same kind of adrenaline rush you do as a player, but as a coach I enjoy the anticipation and excitement in the air before a game and I relish the excitement of the contest itself. And the bigger the contest, the more I enjoy it. I also like being the underdog, which the Broncos were against the 2-0 Wolf Pack.

It's amazing what a football team can do when everybody is "up" and in sync. That was the atmosphere that permeated our club as we took the field against Nevada. In the early moments of the game, each player was swept along in the exhilaration of it all, playing better than he could even imagine. Then we got the capacity crowd roaring and rocking in the opening moments with a perfectly executed 47-yard fleaflicker that went for a touchdown on our first possession. On that play Hilde gave the ball to Adams, who handed off to Ryan Ikebe for an apparent reverse. But Ikebe pitched the ball back to Hilde, who reared back and hurled a long pass to a wide-open Hausske in the end zone. On Nevada's next possession, defensive back Rashid Gayle picked off a pass by quarterback Mike Maxwell and returned it 87 yards to the Wolf Pack one, where Adams scored moments later for a quick 14-0 lead. Before the opening quarter was over, Greg Erickson kicked a 35-yard field goal and Adams scored on a 26-yard run for a stunning 24-0 lead.

But then Nevada got itself straightened out, which I knew it would. You know, sometimes it's scary when you get off to such an early lead against an opponent that is obviously better than you because you know that team is going to come back with a vengeance and make a game out of it; that's exactly what happened. The Wolf Pack scored two touchdowns and a field goal in the second quarter to slice our lead to 24-17. But then we pulled off another spectacular play in the closing seconds of the first half to regain the momentum. With the ball at the Nevada 37, Hilde hit wide receiver Michael Richmond with an eight-yard pass; just as Richmond was about to be tackled, he lateraled the ball to a streaking Adams, who raced 29 yards for his third score of the half and a 31-17 halftime lead.

We couldn't move the ball at all in the third quarter while Nevada scored 10 unanswered points to cut our lead to 31-27; again we were holding on for dear life. Erickson kicked a 19-yard field goal early in the final period to give us a little breathing room at 34-27, but Nevada was still within a touchdown and an extra point of tying the game.

There were plenty of heroics that night, but the thing I remember most was Hilde's gutty performance late in the fourth quarter as we struggled to hold Nevada at bay. The Wolf Pack defense was putting all kinds of pressure on Hilde in a desperate attempt to get the ball back in the final minutes. But Tony made three or four spectacular runs—breaking tackles, spinning away from defenders, refusing to panic—that eventually got us in field goal range and allowed Erickson to ice the game with a 29-yarder in the final minute and a half, giving us a 37-27 upset victory. It was during that game that I knew we had the makings of an outstanding team—and a sophomore quarterback who was something special. Gayle, who would earn first-team All-America honors at the end of the season, was equally spectacular on defense with two interceptions, 12 tackles and a pair of deflections. The Wolf Pack's comeback was no fluke; Nevada went on to post a 9-2 record that year and didn't drop another game until its season finale, a 32-27 setback to UNLV.

After our exciting win over Nevada, we got a bit of a breather the following week with our fourth straight home game—a 35-7 triumph over Liberty University and coach Sam Rutigliano. Hilde threw for three touchdowns and ran for a fourth as we improved to 4-0.

Our first road game was in Flagstaff against Northern Arizona; we came out flat, committed a turnover to start the game, and quickly fell behind 14-0. But Tom Mason's defense was outstanding the rest of the night and Hilde threw second-quarter TD passes to Hausske (22 yards) and Ikebe (29) to forge a 14-14 tie at halftime. After a scoreless third quarter Adams scored on runs of eight and 80 yards in the final period as we won 28-16. We didn't play well against the Lumberjacks that night, but I was encouraged by the fact we still found a way to win. The following week we returned to Bronco Stadium and improved to 6-0 with a 24-17 win over Weber State as Hilde threw touchdown passes to Hausske, Ikebe and tight end Randy Matyshock.

We finally came down to earth in Pocatello the following weekend as Idaho State rallied from a 15-point deficit in the final 18 minutes to hand us a 32-31 loss in Holt Arena. It was a weird game that we should have won. We didn't play well on defense, but our offense moved the ball all night. Erickson had staked us to a 31-16 lead with a 34-yard field goal midway through the third period, and it seemed like we were in control. But the Bengals scored a touchdown late in the third quarter and a field goal midway through the fourth to close to 31-25. Then some really weird stuff started happening.

With a minute remaining in the game we punted the ball deep into Bengal territory. During last-minute situations in close games I try to talk to the players going onto the field to make sure they understand their assignments and know what to watch for. But as I started to walk over to our defensive unit to give our players their last-minute instructions, I saw the ISU punt returner fumble the ball and one of our players recover it. Assuming we had the ball, I turned away from the defense and started talking to Borges and getting our "victory" offense together to run out the clock. Then all at once the officials ruled that ISU had maintained possession because the punt returner had a foot on the sideline and was out-of-bounds when he bobbled the ball. Suddenly, our defensive unit was taking the field before Tom Mason and I had a chance to say anything. But since Idaho State had the ball on its own 13-yard line and no timeouts with just 53 seconds remaining, I didn't think we were in big trouble. Turned out I was wrong.

Our defense screwed up on the very next play as Bengal quarterback Rob Wetta threw a 65-yard pass to Rommie Wheeler to our 22-yard line. After two incompletions Wetta fired a touchdown pass to Kirk Clifford in the back corner of the end zone, and the extra point gave ISU the one-point win in the closing seconds. We blew it; our six-game winning streak was history. And I was pissed. "There's nothing more I hate than losing to a team you're better than," I told Mike Prater of the *Statesman* after the game. "The magic is over. We beat ourselves with a thousand mistakes. ... We learned a hard lesson tonight. I hope the guys can find a way to make use of it because we have some tough football games ahead of us." Never one to mask his emotions or mince his words, defensive end Joe O'Brien had established himself as one of the team's more vocal leaders, and a bit of a clairvoyant. "This team will bounce back," he said to Prater after the game. "We'll work our butts off ... and we'll sweep the rest of our games."

I would have preferred to have beaten the Bengals, but I guess we needed a wake-up call. "Though they didn't like it at the time, the Bronco coaches are in agreement now that the game that turned an interesting but mistake-prone team into a great team was the Idaho State contest," the *Statesman's* Art Lawler later wrote. "Against Idaho State ... the Broncos finally learned the reason they had to take care of business after absorbing a 32-31 loss in the last 20 seconds."

After our setback to the Bengals, we went on a roll. Mason's defense was playing well, Borges' offense was moving the ball, and we rarely made dumb mistakes or committed foolish penalties. For the remainder of the season we played well, we played hard—and most important we played smart. I think our loss to ISU helped us realize that our talent was good but not great; and in order to win, our performance each Saturday had to be predicated on hard-nosed, mistake-free football.

The following week in Bozeman we raced to a 31-3 halftime lead and trounced Montana State 38-10 as Hilde ran for a touchdown and threw for three more and Adams rushed for 103 yards to go over the 1,000-yard mark.

Our next game was at home against unbeaten and top-ranked Montana and Dave Dickenson, the Grizzlies' junior All-America quarterback. Dickenson is a rare kid like Hilde, a competitor who simply refuses to give an inch and will do whatever it takes to win, and his ability to win was nothing short of phenomenal. His record as the starting quarterback for C.M. Russell High School in Great Falls was 24-0. As a sophomore for Montana in 1993, his lone loss was a 49-48 setback to Delaware in the opening round of the Division I-AA playoffs. And entering our game on November 5, Dickenson had led UM to an 8-0 mark, including an impressive 45-21 victory over Idaho the previous week. As a starter in high school and college, he was an astounding 42-1. With Dickenson at quarterback and All-American Scott Gragg—who now starts for the NFL's New York Giants—at offensive tackle, I thought we would have our hands full trying to stop the Grizzlies' potent offense. I mean, Don Read's team was on a *serious* roll. Montana was riding a 15-game conference winning streak and had dropped but two games in its previous 25 contests. With a quarterback of Dickenson's immense talent directing a wide-open offense like Montana's, our coaching staff knew we had to do something drastic to keep him off balance.

Football games are won by players, not coaches. I try to coach every game perfectly and try not to allow any coaching decisions to be the deciding factor between winning and losing. I'm fully aware that once a game begins, the action that transpires on the field is beyond my control. As coaches, all we can do is prepare our players physically and emotionally and hope for the best once the game begins. And to beat Montana, my assistants and I felt we would need the same kind of emotional effort from our team that we had against Nevada. But we also needed to make some tactical adjustments. Fortunately, we had a bye on October 29 and got an extra week to prepare for Dickenson and the Grizzlies. Tom Mason and I knew it was a gamble, but we figured we had to blitz Dickenson in order to have a chance to win. It shouldn't have come as a surprise to Dickenson; after all, I told him what we were going to do four months earlier.

In July of 1994 I was in Missoula on my way to Flathead Lake and stopped in Stockman's Bar, one of the major hangouts for UM sports fans, when I ran into Dickenson and Matt Wells, the Grizzlies' star wide receiver. They greeted me warmly and we engaged in some friendly banter. But given the fact Dickenson had thrown four TD passes in Montana's 38-24 triumph over BSU the previous fall, they definitely had the upper hand. "You guys better be ready when you come down to Boise in November," I said good-naturedly. "You whipped us pretty good up here, but next time we're gonna be blitzing you." We shared a few stories and had a couple of laughs, but I was serious about the blitzing.

And we just happened to have some people who could blitz. They came at Dickenson in waves—13 quarterback sacks for minus-98 yards as we knocked Dickenson out of commission and won 38-14 in what the *Statesman's* Lawler called "a memorable, near-perfect performance." Linebacker Brian Smith led the way with five sacks and nine tackles as our defense punished Dickenson all afternoon—to the point where I almost felt sorry for him in the fourth quarter. Our offense was just as impressive as Hilde threw for 286 yards and three TD passes, two to Ikebe and one to Hausske.

Late in the contest with the game out of reach for Montana, Dickenson suffered a torn tendon in his ankle when he was tackled following a long run along the sidelines. He missed the final two games of the regular season but returned to lead the Grizzlies to a 23-20 first-round playoff victory over Northern Iowa, only to reinjure his leg the following week in UM's 30-28 quarterfinal victory over McNeese State. If Dickenson hadn't messed up his ankle against us on November 5, I think we might have met Montana instead of Youngstown State in the Division I-AA national championship game. Without Dickenson at quarterback, the Grizzlies lost to YSU 28-9 in the semifinals. Sure, Youngstown State had a great club that year, but Montana was not the same team with Dickenson on the sidelines; I think he would have made the difference for the Grizzlies.

But enough about Dickenson; our own star quarterback was injured in that game. Although only a few people realized it at the time, Hilde hurt his shoulder pretty bad against Montana and was never the same. On that day, we were a very good football team as we entered the stretch run for Boise State's first Big Sky championship in 14 years. But the injuries were beginning to take their toll.

Because we had been pointing to our November 19 game with Idaho all season, our coaching staff was worried that we might look past our next opponent—Eastern Washington. Assuming Idaho would beat Weber State on November 12, which it did 79-30, we knew we needed to defeat the Eagles in Cheney that same day to match the Vandals' 5-1 league record and set the stage for a showdown for the conference championship the following week in Boise. Mathematically, we could lose to EWU and still claim the Big Sky's automatic Division I-AA playoff berth by beating Idaho on November 19. But that scenario would technically make us league co-champs with the Vandals, and we wanted the title outright.

Our coaching staff knew the field in EWU's Woodward Stadium was going to be a quagmire, which we found quite worrisome because we were used to playing on artificial turf. But thanks to, um, a fortunate coincidence the week before our game in Cheney, the Boise Fire Department just happened (wink, wink) to be flushing out the fire hydrants near our grass practice field adjacent to the north end of Bronco Stadium. The water from the hydrant had to go *somewhere* (nudge, nudge) and so a few hundred gallons of water ended up on our practice field, creating our own mud bowl and simulating the sloppy conditions we expected to find in Cheney. Around that same time I noticed that a soreness in my upper right arm, which I thought was from a pulled muscle, was getting worse and that a lump had formed in that area. I was also starting to feel sick and listless.

But my ailing body didn't prevent me from having some fun that week. In an attempt to illustrate our team's need to prepare for a muddy confrontation with EWU, the other coaches and I gathered the players around the largest mud puddle on the field following our Wednesday practice session. "OK," Barry Sacks shouted. "Here's how you play in the mud." And he proceeded to dive into the puddle. Then another coach dove in. Then I took off my jacket and shirt, backed up a few steps, ran forward and dived headfirst into the muck. It wasn't a very smart thing to do because I landed awkwardly on my side and found out later that I had cracked a rib. But the point had been made. "Pokey saw it as a motivational tool," Al Borges later told a writer. "I mean, when a 51-year-old head coach dives headfirst into a puddle of mud in the middle of November, how can a player not want to play for a guy like that?" The next day the players got into the act and performed a variety of dives into the mud puddle. It was a fun and unique way to build team unity, but I doubt the people who had to wash our practice uniforms found it very amusing.

A few weeks earlier during a coaches' meeting I remember discussing our receiving corps with Borges. Ikebe had established himself as our top pass catcher while Lee Schrack and Hausske were alternating at the other wideout spot. "We can't alternate them anymore; Hausske simply makes too many big plays," Borges said. "Every game he's in, he makes two or three big-time catches in key situations. We have to play him; we'll use Schrack in our three- and four-receiver formations." I couldn't argue.

Borges' good judgment was never more evident than in the final minutes of our game against Eastern Washington. With 4:09 left we had the ball on our own eight-yard line and trailed 13-9. In one of the more memorable drives in BSU history, Hilde, with the help of three clutch receptions by Hausske, guided our offense 92 yards through the muck and mud of Woodward Stadium. First, Hilde and Hausske teamed for a 26-yard reception to give us some breathing room at our own 34. Later, on a third-and-10, they combined for a 26-yard gain to the EWU 24. A few moments later, again on third-and-10, Hilde hit Hausske with an 18-yard pass to the Eagles' six-yard line, which set up a three-yard touchdown run by Hilde and gave us a 16-13 lead with just over a minute remaining. But the excitement wasn't over yet.

On the ensuing kickoff, Eastern Washington's Jason Anderson broke free for a 37-yard return to the Boise State 43. In the closing seconds Eagle quarterback Todd Bernett quickly drove the EWU offense to our 10-yard line, and after a timeout with three seconds remaining Eastern Washington lined up to try a game-tying field goal, which would send the contest into overtime. But defensive lineman Chris Shepherd blocked Tom Zurfluh's kick to preserve the win. In 1992 Shepherd was perhaps BSU's best defensive lineman, but he suffered a serious knee injury in the second week of the '93 season and was never the same. Despite his limited playing time in 1994, Shepherd twice made his presence felt by blocking field goal attempts—the first time was in our season opener against Northeastern—that would have allowed the opposition to tie the game in the fourth quarter. I was more relieved than happy following our win in Cheney; I had never been so exhausted in my life. And I didn't know why.

Thanks to Shepherd's blocked kick and the clutch play of Hilde and Hausske, our sixth-ranked ballclub entered the final week of the regular season in a position to accomplish the goal we had set for ourselves several months earlier. Our next opponent: archrival Idaho. At stake: the Big Sky title and an automatic berth in the Division I-AA national playoffs. And to add fuel to the fire, Joe O'Brien publicly guaranteed a victory over the Vandals.

IT WAS NO coincidence that Idaho's 12-year dominance over Boise State began when current Seattle Seahawks coach Dennis Erickson took over as the Vandals' head coach in 1982. From Erickson to Keith Gilbertson to John L. Smith, Idaho had been led by three outstanding coaches who deftly guided the school's football program to national prominence in the Division I-AA ranks. (Idaho joined the Division I-A Big West along with BSU in 1996.) And much of that reputation had been forged at Boise State's expense.

I know the University of Idaho always gets cranked up for its game against Boise State, but I think some UI people take the rivalry too seriously. Sure, Boise has its share of rabid Bronco fans, but Boise residents and BSU students do not seem as obsessed with the rivalry as do our counterparts to the north. I think those attitudes reflect the natures of the two cities and schools. Moscow is primarily a college town, and UI has a more traditional student body, complete with an active fraternity and sorority system. Boise on the other hand is a progressive city, and BSU is an urban university with a student population primarily composed of commuters whose daily activities are not directly tied to the campus.

That's not to say the losing streak wasn't a sore spot with BSU football fans. Sure, my assistants and I were well aware of BSU's dozen years of futility and the resentment and frustration the losing streak had created. But you know what? The other coaches and I didn't consider the streak a monkey on our backs. Of those 12 losses, only one belonged to us. Besides, by the end of the 1994 season, we honestly thought our team would finally put an end to the streak—despite the fact the Vandals were 9-1 and ranked third among the nation's Division I-AA teams.

One reason for our optimism was our staff's overall record in the second half of the season. I can't explain why, but for some reason our teams usually played better in the later stages of the season. Going into our game with the Vandals, someone came up with an interesting statistic: If you were to throw out our staff's first season at both PSU and BSU, our overall record for the final five games of the regular campaign at the two schools was 29-6.

Even so, I wasn't overwrought at the prospect of losing to Idaho. Games that we are *expected* to win are the ones that really scare me. Just like Nevada and Montana, I thought Idaho had better talent than we did. In fact, I considered the Vandals the best team in the league that year talentwise. I mean, they had *six* All-Americans including running back Sherriden May, tackle Jim Mills, wide receiver Kyle Gary and defensive end Ryan Phillips. What we had, I thought, was the better *team*. And for the first time in more than a decade, we probably had the better quarterback in Tony Hilde.

Since Idaho began its winning streak in 1982, the Vandal offense had been led by the likes of Ken Hobart, Scott Linehan, John Freisz and Doug Nussmeier, outstanding quarterbacks who were routinely among the best in the Division I-AA ranks—if not the nation. In fact, Freisz and Nussmeier won the NCAA Division I-AA Player of the Year award in 1989 and 1993, respectively, and both are now in the NFL. Vandal QB Brian Brennan was a capable signal caller, but he was only a redshirt freshman; compared to Nussmeier and Freisz, his immediate predecessors, he had a long way to go.

In front of a Bronco Stadium record crowd of 23,701, we squared off with the Vandals in one of the biggest games in the history of the rivalry. Tom Mason had come up with some excellent defensive schemes, which we needed because our offense was starting to struggle. We had some blitz and no-blitz plays we would call based on UI's backfield formation. The previous week against Weber State, the Vandal offense had erupted for 51 points in the first half alone. But Mason's package worked to perfection in the first two quarters as we held Idaho's potent offense to 67 total yards. On offense, Hilde hit Ikebe with a 17-yard touchdown pass and Greg Erickson kicked a pair of field goals to stake us to a 13-0 halftime lead. But much like the Nevada game, I knew we were in for a dogfight in the second half.

At halftime John L. Smith and his staff made some excellent adjustments and UI came storming back. Brennan threw a 73-yard TD pass to tight end Avery Griggs (Brian Smith blocked the PAT) and Ryan

Woolverton added a 25-yard field goal to cut our lead to 13-9. Hilde and Ikebe then hooked up for an 11-yard TD pass late in the third period to increase our lead to 20-9. But Brennan brought Idaho to within 20-17 with another huge scoring play—an 82-yard bomb to Gary, the Big Sky's leading receiver who was held to two catches that day. But Hilde and our offense responded by moving the ball 75 yards in four plays, and Tony and Ikebe combined for their third TD of the game, a 45-yard strike, for a 27-17 lead. The Vandals scored a TD with just over two minutes left, and tried an onside kick on the ensuing play. But Hausske caught the ball and we held on for the 27-24 win.

The place went nuts. BSU had its first Big Sky title since 1980 and earned its first berth in the I-AA playoffs since 1990. Most important to many Bronco fans, the streak was over. Hundreds of fans descended from the stands and spilled onto the field to celebrate the win—letting loose after a dozen years of pent-up frustration. "This is the greatest moment of my life!" declared Joe O'Brien. "I backed up my words. No, this team backed up my words!"

Our game plan worked much like it did against Nevada: Surprise the hell out of the opposition with some new wrinkles on defense, hope to pull off some big plays on offense, and hold on for dear life. "We were taking heavy risks on defense, but it worked out," I told the media after the game.

"When you blitz, sometimes you get burned and we gave up a couple of long passes," Mason added. "But we felt comfortable with the players we had out there on the field. They knew the system."

Hilde had an outstanding game, but he was really hurting afterward. K.C. Adams was also banged up and had started to lose some of his effectiveness. I don't want to make excuses, but like I said, we were never the same physically after the Montana game. And I wasn't feeling so good myself. I remember standing near the middle of the field at the end of the game, enjoying the whole scene and watching Al Borges climb up on the north-end goalpost with the fans. But I also remember how exhausted I felt at that moment. That night I went out and celebrated with some friends, including my sister and her husband. But I can remember asking Jennie and Jack to drive me home before midnight because I was just too tired to stay out any longer. And that wasn't my style.

My weariness was starting to worry me. Other than the soreness in my arm, I didn't feel sick per se—just kind of weird and tired all the time. I just attributed it to the stress of the season and the inner turmoil related to my separation from Barb. "Jeez, I feel like shit," I said to Mason a few days later as we prepared for our playoff opener against North Texas. "What's the deal? Maybe I'm just getting old."

SPEAKING OF PERSONAL problems, I found it quite ironic that all of a sudden my private life was coming under media scrutiny as we began to win. In fact, during the final month or so of the 1994 season I had two or three Boise television reporters apologize to me for the snooping their stations had been doing into my private life. It seemed someone had started a rumor that I had been charged with driving under the influence, and somebody called the Boise TV stations to fan the flames of that rumor. I know at least two of the local stations sent a reporter to the Ada County Prosecutor's Office to check it out. By that time it was also pretty well known that Barb and I had separated and she had moved to Missoula, so someone also started a rumor that she left because I had been beating her. And again, at least one station sent a reporter to the prosecutor's office to check if I had ever been charged with assault.

We had a bye the week between the Montana State and the Montana games, and I was in Los Angeles during that time on a recruiting trip when Jerry Jones, a reporter from Boise TV station KTVB, called me in L.A. "Pokey," he said, "I just want to apologize."

"What are you talking about?" I said.

"Well, my sources said that you had a DUI, so we had to check it and we were down at the prosecutor's office and from everything I could find out, you don't have one."

"For chrissakes, I could have told you that! You should have called me before you checked. Who are your sources?"

"I can't tell you."

Gee … how convenient. I guess it's OK for people to lie about me, but when I ask who my accusers are, their anonymity is protected.

Then when I got back to Boise, Dana Haynes from KIVI Channel 6 called me. "Pokey, she said, "I feel really bad about this."

"Bad about what?" I said.

"My news director told me to go to the prosecutor's office, and spend all day if necessary looking through files. We heard that not only do you have a DUI, but that your wife filed an assault charge against you. These rumors are unsubstantiated, but I've gotta do my job and check them out."

Later I heard about another whopper: Not only did I get the assault charge expunged from the records, but some big booster paid the fine and gave Barbara $50,000 to leave town.

Sick. Vicious. Unbelievable. It was almost too much to handle. It makes me angry to have to defend myself against such ridiculous and base- less accusations, but for the record: I have never had a DUI and I have never struck my wife. In fact, when I called Barb in Missoula and told her about the "charges," she laughed and said, "Hey, for $50,000 I'll fly down and let you slap me; then we can split the money."

A FOOTBALL PLAYER with one hand? A kicker, sure. An offensive line- man, maybe. But a *defensive back*? Sure, DaWuan Miller could run the 40- yard dash in under five seconds and bench press 300 pounds. Great. But what about that missing appendage? It was no problem for the three-year starter, who in 1994 led our defense in passes broken up with 16. Miller was born with a left arm that ended at the elbow, but his disability had little bearing on his athletic prowess. As a high school senior in Battle Ground, Washington, he rushed for more than 1,000 yards, scored eight touchdowns, made 48 tackles, and intercepted four passes in only eight games. He also starred in baseball and basketball and was an honor stu- dent.

"Catching a football was not complex," said reporter Tom Friend, who wrote a feature on DaWuan for the *New York Times* in early Decem- ber of 1994. "He extends for the ball like anyone with two hands would. He uses his right fingers for squeezing and his nub for supporting. 'I've never had a left hand, so I don't know any other way,' Miller said. He throws his hard body at running backs to tackle them, although his posi- tion coach, Ron Gould, advises him to 'grab cloth if he can.'"

Miller was the only freshman starter on Skip Hall's defense in 1992; in 1993 he made 30 tackles and had two interceptions. Even so, opposing teams still tended to throw the ball his way to test his perceived handi- cap. Big mistake, as North Texas would learn in the first round of the Di- vision I-AA playoffs. Much like the situation at Portland State, BSU, which had risen to No. 3 in the final Division I-AA poll, could all but guarantee a capacity crowd for any playoff game it hosted; thus we got the home-field advantage in our opening-round game against 18th-ranked UNT. With the exception of our blowout victories over Liberty and Montana State, every game that season was a tight, tense, hard-fought struggle; the script would remain the same in the playoffs.

Hilde hit Ikebe with a 40-yard touchdown pass and Erickson kicked a 29-yard field goal in the first quarter, but the Eagles scored two TDs and two field goals in the first half to take a 20-10 lead at the intermission. After a scoreless third period, a spectacular 35-yard reception by Hausske at the Eagles' goal line set up a one-yard TD run by Adams midway through the fourth quarter to make it 20-17.

On North Texas' ensuing possession, Eagle quarterback Mitch Maher was faced with a third-and-eight situation deep in his own territory. Maher faded back and lofted a pass over the middle, where DaWuan Miller was waiting. Miller dashed in front of the intended receiver, "used his one and a half arms to intercept" the pass, the *Times'* Friend wrote, and returned it to the UNT six-yard line. On the next play Hilde hit running back Willie Bowens in the end zone with 5:38 remaining for the game-winning score and a 24-20 triumph. "In lieu of a consistent [offensive] attack, a wild, gambling defense came up with several big plays to keep the Broncos' playoff hopes alive," wrote the *Statesman's* Lawler after the season. "None was bigger than Miller's interception."

Lawler was right. With a rash of injuries to key players, our offense was struggling. Fortunately, our defense had been playing well since the Idaho State game. Led by linebacker Brian Smith, who had 20 tackles against UNT, we held the Eagles scoreless in the second half to post the win and advance to the quarterfinals against Appalachian State.

The toll that the long season had taken on our offensive unit was never more evident than the following Saturday in Bronco Stadium as the 17th-ranked Mountaineers held us to zero yards total offense in the opening quarter. In fact, with the exception of a couple of huge plays by Hilde and Ikebe, our offense had trouble all afternoon, losing three fumbles and giving up four interceptions. Hilde's shoulder was really hurting him while Adams (shoulder and ankle), Ikebe (shoulder) and Hausske (leg) were all banged up. In addition, Paul Coffman, our first-team All-Big Sky center, didn't play against Appalachian State because of a shoulder injury.

Despite our offensive woes, Hilde hit Ikebe with a 61-yard touchdown pass and Greg Erickson kicked a 45-yard field goal in the second quarter as we grabbed a 10-7 lead at halftime. Then our defense bailed us out again, holding ASU scoreless in the third quarter while Hilde and Ikebe combined for another huge play—a 64-yard TD pass late in the third quarter—to extend our lead to 17-7. Our defense, led by Stefan Reid's 17 tackles and 13 more by Travis Thompson, was outstanding. We held ASU to 226 total yards, allowing the Mountaineers to complete just seven of 27 passing attempts for 73 yards as we advanced to the semifinals with a 17-14 win.

But we were lucky. I didn't think we could play another game like that and expect to win. Like I said, I thought we were a great football team when we beat Montana. But the injuries were beginning to mount. Hilde continued to make the big play, but he was never the same after our win over the Grizzlies. I think our wins over North Texas and Appalachian State were just a matter of will. We had become used to winning, we had formed good habits, we had good workouts; we found ways to win with luck and pluck.

In the summer of 1996 *FOCUS*, Boise State's alumni magazine, printed a list of the 10 greatest moments in BSU sports history during the school's 26 years in the Big Sky. In the article, the magazine's editors had our Division I-AA semifinal game against second-ranked Marshall University on the list, simply calling it "The Comeback."

"It was the crowning moment of a glorious season," the article read. "It was an improbable comeback in a season full of comebacks against a formidable foe that looked unstoppable." Indeed Marshall, 12-1 and the 1993 national runner-up, had us on the ropes in the first half in our December 10 game in Bronco Stadium. We seemed hopelessly behind as the Thundering Herd twice led by 17 points in the second quarter. And our situation became even bleaker when Hilde reinjured his bad shoulder after being tackled in the final two minutes of the half with Marshall ahead 24-7. But then we rallied, as we had done all year. Backup quarterback Mark Paljetak, who had thrown a total of four passes all season, entered the game and promptly marched our offense 61 yards in five plays, hitting Lee Schrack with a screen pass for a 34-yard touchdown with less than a minute remaining before halftime. Suddenly, surprisingly, we were trailing only 24-14 at the intermission; our club and the more than 20,000 fans in Bronco Stadium were back in the game.

I wasn't even going to let Hilde leave the locker room in the second half. But after checking with the team doctors, Al Borges told me Tony could play if necessary. I decided, however, to stay with Paljetak to start the third quarter. But our offense sputtered to open the second half as Adams lost a fumble and Paljetak threw an interception, so I decided to reinsert Hilde late in the third quarter. Tony engineered an 89-yard drive that cut Marshall's lead to 24-21 with a two-yard TD by Adams early in the fourth quarter.

And while our offense was chipping away at Marshall's lead, our defense was stopping the Thundering Herd cold. Marshall had seven possessions in the second half; twice they turned the ball over on downs and the other five drives ended in punts. With about nine minutes remaining in regulation, our defense forced Marshall to punt and our offense took over on the Thundering Herd's 45. Three plays later Hilde hit Schrack with a 34-yard TD pass for a 28-24 lead with 7:51 remaining. Our defense held, but the game wasn't decided until Keith Walk-Green batted down Marshall quarterback Todd Donnan's desperation pass in the end zone on the final play of the game. With our amazing comeback victory, Boise State advanced to the Division I-AA national championship game for the first time since 1980.

"This team truly makes the plays when it has to," I said afterward. "It's amazing. I didn't know what to expect today, but I knew this team wouldn't quit. Everybody talks about magic and destiny and all that stuff, but let me tell you this: We've got to be an awfully good football team to come back from 24-7 and win against a team like Marshall."

It was luck, it was spirit, it was the home-field advantage through the first three games. All those ingredients helped us make it to the title game, but the primary reason for our success—and I know it's a cliché—was because our players and coaches cared about each other. We stuck together and continued to beat teams that were probably more talented. I was amazed, but I also had serious doubts if our so-called magic could continue for one more game.

OUR OFFENSE HAD taken a severe beating over the course of the previous 15 weeks. Doctors said Hilde's shoulder would require surgery after the season, but I was also told he couldn't hurt it any worse and could play in the national championship game the following week against Youngstown State, which had defeated Montana 28-9 in the other semifinal contest. In addition, I was having serious concerns about my own health.

Starting with our double sessions in August, I had been trying to work out all season. I started doing two sets of 15 push-ups and 30 sit-ups, increasing those numbers each week. By mid-October I was doing two sets of 45 push-ups and 100 sit-ups. I don't remember the exact date, but I was feeling good one particular day as I was doing my push-ups in the Varsity Center weight room after practice, so I figured what the hell, I'll just go for a nice round figure of 50.

The next morning while I was driving to work, I had this pain in my upper right arm. "God, my arm hurts," I remember saying to Barry Sacks. "I must have pulled a muscle in my triceps with those extra five push-ups." I didn't think much of it after that, but my arm continued to bother me the rest of the season. I later felt a lump in my arm, but I figured it was a pulled or ruptured muscle. It didn't seem like a big deal at the time.

Around the same time, I started feeling, well, old. On Saturday nights after a home game our staff usually goes out to unwind, and we've been known to stay out pretty late—especially when we're winning like we were that fall. I'm certainly one who enjoys socializing after a game, but by the end of the season I wasn't in much of a mood to party—despite our amazing success. And when I did go out, it wasn't the same. Barb and I had separated by then, but I felt so fatigued I didn't even feel like being with women.

Meanwhile, the pain in my arm would not abate, so I talked to Gary Craner, our head trainer, but he couldn't figure out what it was. I mentioned my discomfort to other people, and they said the same thing: It was probably just a pulled muscle or maybe a calcium deposit. One of our team doctors said I should just stretch my arm because I probably had some muscle mass knotted up in the triceps and needed to work it loose. But after I tried that, I think I popped some blood vessels around the tumor because the swelling increased and the pain had become constant. By the time we played North Texas in the first round of the playoffs, I was really miserable. But I just figured it was the result of the long, stressful season and my marital problems.

Making good on a promise I had made if 20,000 fans showed up for the Marshall game, I rode on horseback for about half a mile to the weekly boosters' luncheon in the BSU Student Union the Monday following our victory over Marshall. All I can remember about that horse ride was how bad I felt. I was in so much pain I finally went to see George Wade, our team physician, that same afternoon.

I could tell right away he was concerned; all of a sudden it wasn't a pulled muscle anymore. "Jiminy Christmas, something's not right here," I remember him saying. He scheduled me for an MRI that same evening.

On Wednesday morning, December 14, just a few hours before we left for Huntington, West Virginia, site of the national championship game, Wade drained blood and some other fluid from the lump and performed a biopsy. He attached a device to my arm to collect the excess blood coming out of the incision and put my arm in a sling. When our team, the rest of the BSU entourage, and the members of the media boarded the chartered plane for the trip to Huntington that afternoon, it was obvious something was wrong with my arm. "Hey, Max," a reporter said to Max Corbet, our sports information director. "What's wrong with Pokey's arm?"

"Oh, he just had a cyst removed," Corbet replied.

Speaking of Huntington, I don't think I got off on the right foot with the folks there. It was bad enough that we had defeated their team and preempted Marshall's plans to play for the national championship in its own stadium, but then I added insult to injury during a live radio broadcast back to West Virginia the morning after our semifinal victory over the Herd. As I sat down for the interview I suddenly realized I had no idea where Marshall was. "Oh man," I said to myself, "I'm really gonna screw this up." Sure enough, I ended up calling the site of the title game "Boonesville," not Huntington. It was a huge gaffe. I mean, I didn't have the school, the city or the state right; I was thinking Appalachian State, which is in Boone, North Carolina.

Anyway, I was really uncomfortable during the flight; needless to say I wasn't my fun-loving self during that trip. But having the lump drained relieved some of the pressure, and my arm felt a little better during the next couple of days in Huntington. I followed Wade's orders during the trip with one exception: I was not going to walk around Huntington and coach our football team with my arm in a sling. Wade said my ailing limb would feel better if I kept it supported, but I got rid of the sling when we got to Huntington because I thought it would draw too much attention; besides I thought it made me look like a wimp. In any case, I really didn't have time to dwell on my physical problems; the quality of our opposition and our team's physical condition gave me enough to worry about.

I wouldn't say Youngstown State—the top-ranked and unbeaten defending national champ—was invincible, but the Penguins were awfully damn good, and our injuries only hurt our chances. Hilde could barely lift his arm above his shoulder and Adams hadn't been a factor in the playoffs because of his assorted injuries. I also felt some personal pressure. This was my third national championship game as a head coach, and having lost the two previous times, I desperately wanted to win this one. Also, BSU had won the national crown in its only other appearance in the title game in 1980, and to merit any comparisons with that great team of Jim Criner's, we would have to beat the Penguins.

I don't know if the players could sense my physical pain and inner turmoil, but I just had the feeling we were in trouble as game day approached. Our team had played hard all season and had ridden an emotional wave through the playoffs. But we also knew we had been extremely lucky to win our three postseason games. In retrospect, I think some of them were hurting so badly that they just wanted to get the season over with. From the moment we arrived in Huntington I had a feeling that the odds were about to catch up with us. A trip to play in a national championship game should have been a fun time, but it wasn't for me. At the Thursday evening banquet for the two teams, the head coaches were supposed to be the featured speakers. But I wasn't up to it. I told Al Borges to take my place, returned to my hotel room and went to bed.

At 13-0-1 and winner of two of the previous three I-AA national championships, Youngstown State was the clear favorite. The Penguins had 23 seniors to our nine and their defense had given up an average of less than 10 points per contest.

In the first few minutes of the nationally televised title game I thought maybe we could establish some momentum because we got off to a reasonably good start. Jermaine Hudson made a fine return of the opening kickoff, bringing the ball to Youngstown State's 41-yard line. Hilde then hit Ikebe with a 15-yard pass to the Penguins' 26. "Hey," I said to Borges on the sidelines, "this is pretty neat!" But on the next two plays Hilde was sacked for a nine-yard loss and we drew a five-yard penalty. After a short run by Hilde, Greg Erickson tried a 51-yard field goal, which fell short. A few minutes later, however, strong safety Chris Cook intercepted a pass by YSU quarterback Mark Brungard and ran it back 58 yards to the Penguins' five. On the next play Hilde hit tight end Randy Matyshock with a pass in the end zone and we had a 7-0 lead.

Perhaps if we had scored on our first series and had a 14-0 or 10-0 lead we might have played with more confidence, but we just finally ran out of gas—emotionally and physically—and didn't play well the rest of the game. Youngstown State, on the other hand, played extremely well. Brungard scored on a two-yard run in the second quarter to tie the game at 7. Then came the turning point. With less than a minute to go before halftime YSU had driven to our 38. We had called for a blitz, and Brungard saw it. He audibled for a quarterback draw, took the snap, dropped back as if to pass, tucked the ball in his arm and raced untouched into the end zone for a touchdown and a 14-7 lead. All season long we had gambled and won on plays like that, but it looked like our good fortune was about to run out. The Penguins scored two more TDs in the second half—the second on a 55-yard run by Shawn Patton—to increase their lead to 28-7 before Hilde hit Matyshock with a six-yard touchdown pass late in the game to make the final score a somewhat respectable 28-14. But YSU was the better team that day. We had only 225 yards total offense.

"In the end, the lack of physically healthy bodies to put on the field had about as much to do with the team's downfall as did a very good Youngstown State team," wrote the *Statesman's* Art Lawler. "The loss showed that even teams with heart can't defy all obstacles. The Penguins repeatedly found Bronco weaknesses and exploited them on both sides of the ball."

It was a pretty sad scene in the locker room, to say the least. Offensive line coach Dave Stromswold was crying and so were a few of the players. I was disappointed, but I wasn't as down as I thought I would be. Of course I wanted to win that last game and bring a national championship back to Boise. But I also knew that we went further than anyone expected us to. Our amazing autumn of 1994 was a product of hard work and dedication—rooted in the abilities of our coaching staff and made possible by a group of players who believed in themselves. Luck, commitment and a passion to win brought the Broncos to the brink of a national championship, but in the end we were just too hobbled to give Youngstown State a real fight. "We were kind of living on borrowed time," I told the media in the postgame press conference. "We had a great run. We hit our peak when we beat Montana. We were healthy and we were really a great football team. But after that point, we became more and more injured. Yet somehow we found a way to win. We ran out of magic. You can only go so far with heart and luck and courage."

"For all their heart and spirit the Broncos were woefully short on healthy 'weapons' throughout the playoffs," Lawler wrote. "Their weekly offensive production fell by about 200 yards a game from the last half of the regular season."

Still, the '94 squad was a team with pizzazz or charisma—whatever you want to call it. It was a real close team with a bunch of outstanding young men who provided Boise State fans with a league championship and one of the most endearing and improbable seasons in school history. The 1994 campaign wasn't simply a successful "rebuilding" year at Boise State—our 13-2 record gave us a school record for victories and the second-best turnaround in I-AA football history. We didn't win the national championship, but that roster was filled with winners.

And there were plenty of individual honors to go around at the end of the season. Defensive end Joe O'Brien and defensive back Rashid Gayle were named first-team All-Americans by the Associated Press and running back K.C. Adams was a second-team selection. O'Brien, Gayle and Adams were also named first-team All-Big Sky along with center Paul Coffman and guard Alex Toyos. O'Brien was named the Big Sky's Defensive MVP and Adams was chosen as Top Newcomer. Ryan Ikebe, Greg Erickson, Brian Smith, Chris Cook and punter Danny Weeks were second-team all-league picks. I was named 1994 Big Sky Coach of the Year and NCAA Division I-AA Region Coach of the Year.

So the storied 1980 team remained Boise State's lone national champ. Well, maybe the 1994 Broncos weren't the school's best team ever, but they sure were a helluva lot of fun.

Chapter 13

Confronting Cancer

Our football team got back to Boise the night of December 17 at around 8. Although I wasn't feeling much better, our coaching staff still had one more rite of passage to fulfill before we could call it a night—and a season. After we got off the plane and back to campus, where we were greeted by a couple hundred fans, the other coaches and I took the seniors—Jarett Hausske, Lee Schrack, Joe O'Brien, Chris Cook, Stefan Reid, et al—to a local establishment a few blocks from Bronco Stadium for a small party to commemorate their careers. Our gathering didn't last long, mostly because I was really feeling bad and just wanted to go to bed.

I knew something was wrong with my arm, but I honestly never gave any thought to the possibility I might have cancer. I just thought the lump in my right triceps was a cyst or something. My pain and fatigue notwithstanding, things had seemingly returned to normal by the following Monday, December 19—a date I won't forget. I was my usual smart-alecky self during my speech at the weekly luncheon of the Bronco Athletic Association, BSU's booster club. "I know I'll probably get in trouble for saying this," I told the crowd. "But I'd rather lose and get to live in Boise than win and have to live in Youngstown, Ohio, any day." The audience roared with laughter and I continued with a few more jokes and one-liners.

But about 30 minutes later, in an examining room in the Idaho Sports Medicine Institute, circumstances dictated a much more serious tone. George Wade, our team physician, told me I had cancer—a rare, insidious, deadly tissue cancer called rhabdomyosarcoma.

I guess I suspected something was up from the way Wade had treated the lump in my triceps during our team's three days in West Virginia; throughout the trip he seemed quite concerned and kept checking the tube he had attached to my upper arm. In fact, as we prepared for the championship game against Youngstown State, he seemed more worried about me than our players.

After I got the bad news from Wade, the next day and a half seemed like a blur. That same afternoon Wade sent me to see Dr. Carolyn Collins, a regional sarcoma cancer expert and director of medical oncology at St. Alphonsus Cancer Treatment Center in Boise who agreed to oversee my treatment. As Collins told me later, it was kind of amusing when Wade set up the appointment.

"I have this fellow who has rhabdo," Wade said.

"Fine," Collins replied, "I'll see him tomorrow."

"It's Pokey Allen."

"Fine, I'll see him tomorrow."

"You know who he is, don't you?"

"No."

"He's the BSU football coach."

"Uh … all right."

"You know, the guy who won all the games this year."

"Um, I really don't follow football."

"He's the guy who rode the horse down Broadway last week."

"Oh, *that* guy."

When I got to St. Al's, Collins ordered all kinds of tests—CAT (computerized axial tomography) scans of my upper chest, abdomen and pelvis; a bone scan; and a bone marrow aspirate and biopsy (a rather uncomfortable procedure in which a long needle is pushed through the skin of the lower back and into the pelvic bone and about a teaspoonful of marrow is drawn out; the marrow is sent to a lab and examined for evidence of cancerous cells). One of the first things I asked Collins was if I could go home to Missoula for Christmas, which was less than a week away. "You can begin your treatment now or you can start when you get back from the holidays," she said. "But I'll tell you something: You never know what is going to happen with this kind of cancer. It's nasty and aggressive; if I were you I wouldn't wait." So I called my mom and explained the situation. Well, shoot, later that week she came down from Missoula, and the rest of my family—my sister and her husband, Jennie and Jack Kirschling, and their two kids, Tara and Ryan—flew down from Seattle to spend Christmas with me in Boise.

Of course I was distressed by the news, but I was surprised how hard it hit many of my friends and colleagues—my roommate Mike Young, for instance. Young, BSU's longtime wrestling coach, moved in with me after my wife and I separated the previous summer, and we eventually bought a town house together. But Mike and I are more than roommates; he's one of my closest friends. When I told him I had cancer, he all of a sudden got tears in his eyes. I was slightly embarrassed and didn't know what to say, so I cussed him out. "Goddamit, Mike," I said. "What are you doing?"

"I don't know," he said. "It just sort of hit me wrong."

"Well, knock it off. You're acting like a goddam woman."

On Tuesday, December 20, I was named Big Sky Coach of the Year. But accolades seemed unimportant now. That same morning I broke the news about my illness to Gene Bleymaier, our athletic director; Max Corbet, our sports information director; my assistant coaches; and other members of the BSU athletic department. Most of our players, however, had already scattered for the Christmas break, so there was no way to inform them. In fact, Martez Benas, one of our starting guards, said he didn't find out about my illness until he heard it on ESPN while he was home in Chicago. Speculation among the Boise media had been brewing because of my arm problems in Huntington, so it was decided to hold a press conference at St. Al's Cancer Treatment Center the next day.

I guess I was still a bit numbed by what had transpired over the previous 48 hours because I don't remember much about the press conference. I do recall being surprised by the large number of reporters who were jammed into that little conference room that morning. I didn't have a prepared statement; I was just there to listen to Collins explain my situation, answer questions, and get it over with. Usually when I make a few wisecracks at a press conference, the laughter is nearly automatic. But when I tried to crack a few jokes this time, nothing but solemn faces stared back at me. It was a strange scene—almost surreal in retrospect. I mean, four days earlier I had been coaching in a national championship game, and now, out of the blue, I was sitting at a press conference disclosing to the world that I had cancer. My treatment, Collins told the reporters, would entail chemotherapy, surgery and radiation that would take about a year.

I told the media I didn't want anyone's pity; I meant it at the time, and I still mean it now as I work on this book in the fall of 1996. People who need pity are those who go through something like this and don't have a support system like mine. I have a great family and many friends whom I can count on. Besides, I've had the best life that anybody has ever had. Sure, I've had some problems along the way, but then who hasn't? Shoot, I've had a great life. I'm going to fight this cancer all the way. But if things don't work out, at least I enjoyed the ride.

Before we faced the media, Collins told me the preliminary results from the tests she had ordered two days earlier showed no indications of cancer in my bones, lymph nodes or vital organs; but she reiterated that rhabdomyosarcoma is a highly aggressive and unpredictable form of cancer and that we should begin the battle right away. So immediately following the press conference I began my first chemotherapy treatment with the introduction of the drugs cyclophosphamide, adriamycin and vincristine into my body.

The only time I got emotional during those first few days was when I phoned my estranged wife, who was living in Montana with our 14-month-old daughter. Despite our impending divorce Barbara and I remained close, and I dreaded having to call her. During our marriage her life had twice been cursed by cancer. Her dad passed away in 1991 and her mom died in 1993, both victims of the disease that now had a grip on me. "Barb, I'm so glad we're separated and getting a divorce now because I don't want you to go through this again," I said. "I don't want you to worry about it. I don't want you to think you have to come back to Boise. You don't have to do anything. Just take care of Taylor, and I can work this out. I have my sister and the rest of my family. Don't change your life. I'm going to beat this."

I wasn't trying to be a martyr. Barb's family is the most important thing in her life, and she had been devastated by the loss of her parents; I honestly didn't want her to have to go through such an ordeal a third time. We cried together on the phone; it was the one time I broke down. At the time, I found it ironic that I had contracted cancer because I knew I could have been more supportive of Barb when her folks were dying. In both cases I never made it to Montana to see them when the end was near because I was too busy coaching. I felt bad that I didn't spend enough time with Barb and help her in her hour of need.

My conversation with Barbara was the one time my emotions got the best of me. On the whole, I've tried to approach my battle with cancer, now going on 22 months, with the same philosophy I've used for the last 20 years: Treat everything as an adventure. When I face difficult situations, such as this cancer, from that point of view, the situation seems somewhat easier for me to handle. After I was diagnosed with cancer, I decided, "Hey, this is something not a lot of people will go through, so let's look at it as an adventure and make the best of the journey." It's kind of interesting when you think about it in those terms. Some people might think this is a strange way to approach a potentially deadly illness, but it seems to work for me. Some people call it a foolish attitude, others say I'm brave. I don't think I'm either; it's just the way I handle adversity.

During the 1994 holiday season I never had morbid thoughts like, "This is my last Christmas" or anything like that. I think it's self-defeating to think in those terms. In fact, my primary concern was my golf game. During the first few days of my treatment, Collins told me I would be undergoing more medical procedures that might preclude me from golfing that spring. Now *that*, I told her, is what I called bad news. But all in all, the holidays that year were not much different than the previous ones.

After my mom and sister returned home a few days after Christmas, I went out on New Year's Eve with my coaches and their wives. It was like nothing had changed; I even had a date. I remember we ended up at Yen Ching, a Chinese restaurant in downtown Boise. But while I was sitting there laughing and talking, I could feel the intravenous access device that was sending chemotherapy drugs into my system. I thought, "Hey, if this is what it's like, no problem. I can get through this."

If only it had all been that painless.

THE BATTERY OF tests and treatments designed to shrink the malignancy in my right triceps and fend off the cancer continued through the first two and a half months of 1995 in Boise. In January I began taking two new chemotherapy drugs, ifosfamide and VP-16, five days a week. Despite the treatments, I still managed to make several recruiting trips from January through March.

Collins said my body was tolerating the chemotherapy drugs just fine, but during a two- or three-day period in mid-January I had become susceptible to bacterial infection because my white blood cell count (the number of cells that fight bacteria) was down to zero. She feared that if I fell victim to fever or infection without a defense system I could possibly get bacteria in my bloodstream and suffer a condition called septic shock, which is potentially fatal. But Collins also had me taking a hormone called G-CSF (granulocyte colony stimulating factor) or neupogen, which helps white cells grow rapidly, and I eventually got by that crisis.

The most obvious side effect to my cancer treatment was the loss of all my hair. But my bald head was the least of my worries. In February Collins determined that the tumor, albeit softer, had not shrunk to her satisfaction; it was "just kind of sitting there, not doing very much," she explained. Both Collins and George Wade recommended that the tumor be surgically removed. After another month of chemotherapy treatment in Boise, I went to the University of Washington Medical Center in Seattle, and on March 16 Dr. Chappie Conrad, Collins' colleague and an oncological orthopedic surgeon who specializes in tumors of the bone and soft tissue, performed a "radical resection of the right triceps." The media always described the tumor in spherical terms—the size of a baseball or a grapefruit. Its shape, however, was more elliptical than bulbous. Rather than a round mass sitting in one spot, the tumor was attached up and down my right triceps muscle. About four inches long and two and a half inches wide, its shape more closely resembled a banana without the pointed ends than a ball. But I really didn't care what it looked like, I was just glad the damned thing was finally out.

But my battle had just begun. Although the operation went well, the long-term prognosis was "not good," Collins told me afterward. She expected as much. Before the operation, doctors did a positive emission tomography, or PET scan, of my upper right arm. The results of the PET scan, an imaging device that provides a metabolic picture of the activity of an area of tissue, did not bode well.

"What we wanted was a dead tumor," Collins explained. "Unfortunately, before you went into the operating room, we had a very strong suspicion that the tumor was alive by virtue of the PET scan." Collins' fears were well-founded. "The tumor was 100 percent viable," she said. "There wasn't a dead cell in it. And that's bad news. Ideally, what we wanted was to see it 100 or 90 percent dead, but 100 percent alive was not good. It means that any tumor cells that may have spread to a lung, your liver, lymph nodes or bone would also potentially be alive."

Conrad's prognosis was equally grim. A day or so after the operation he visited me in my hospital room. "Dr. Conrad," I said, "I'm in trouble, aren't I?"

"I'm afraid so," he answered. "It's not a good sign to have the tumor still viable. The normal procedure would be to return to the chemotherapy treatment, but it obviously didn't kill the cancer cells in the tumor."

"So, if you were me, what would you do?"

"I would suggest you think about a stem-cell transplant."

I recovered well after the surgery, returned to Boise a few days later, and was on hand when our spring practices began the following month. The side effects of my cancer treatment, however, did force me to miss the last five practice sessions, if I remember correctly. It was the first time in my 10 years as a head coach that I ever missed a practice or a game. Being back on the football field boosted my morale considerably, but in regard to my long-term survival, Collins said there was little reason for optimism. In late March, after consulting several colleagues, including fellow sarcoma cancer specialists in Houston and Seattle, Collins concurred with Conrad's recommendation and told me that a stem-cell transplant was probably my best, if not my only, hope for long-term survival. There were no totally reliable statistics to predict my chances, the doctor said, but she and her fellow cancer experts agreed that to proceed as they had been with standard therapy would give me only a 10 to 15 percent chance of still being alive in five years. Alarmingly, my chances had significantly *decreased* from the 40 to 60 percent odds I was given when I began my treatment three months earlier. A stem-cell transplant combined with high doses of chemotherapy *might* improve those odds to around 30 percent, Collins said. But the side effects inherent in such a procedure, she warned me, are themselves life-threatening.

"What you would be doing by selecting the transplant option," Collins said to me, "is taking a tremendous risk in the short term for having *only the potential* for long-term survival." The conversation that followed was brief: "So if I don't do anything, this cancer is probably going to kill me, right?" I asked.

"That's right," Collins replied.

"And if I have this transplant done and the *treatment* doesn't kill me, I have a better chance of living?"

"Maybe."

"Then let's do it."

Part of the reason that I agreed to the stem-cell transplant was because I thought the time frame delineated by Collins—assuming everything went according to plan—would allow me enough time to undergo the treatment, recover sufficiently and be back in Boise by early August to prepare for the 1995 football season. Had I been diagnosed with cancer during another time of year, I would have forgone the stem-cell transplant; I wasn't going to miss football merely to increase my chances by 15 percent.

In April the procedure to harvest stem cells from my blood began at Boise's other hospital, St. Luke's Regional Medical Center, in preparation for a stem-cell transplant at Seattle's Fred Hutchinson Cancer Research Center. Combined with aggressive chemotherapy, the process eventually wiped out my white blood cells and touched off a series of medical crises that, among other complications, triggered several episodes of an irregular heartbeat and weakened my immune system to the point that I was twice near death, though I didn't realize it at either time.

The first time was on April 14, Good Friday, at St. Al's. I had driven myself to the hospital because I had a feeling something was seriously wrong. Collins initially thought I might be going into septic shock (I wasn't), and I was admitted immediately. I remember lying in a small room waiting for Collins while an attending nurse was periodically taking my pulse and blood pressure. While I was waiting, my blood pressure dropped from 85/50 to 65/30 and my pulse dropped from 60 to 40 in a matter of minutes. Then I heard somebody yell, "Code blue!" and all of a sudden I was surrounded by five doctors and six nurses sticking IVs in me, giving me oxygen and acting like something was seriously wrong.

I think they thought I was having a heart attack; my heart was not pumping the blood or some damn thing, I'm not really sure. But the funny thing was that while I was lying there, I didn't feel any different than I had two or three hours earlier. I was conscious the whole time and never felt like my life was in danger. I just felt tired and weak. As Collins and the others feverishly worked to stabilize my condition, I looked up at Collins and said, "You know, it was a good thing I watched *ER* last night, because I kind of know what's going on here now." Collins chuckled and replied, "Only you would say something like that."

My condition was diagnosed as an irregular heartbeat called brady-cardia and I was placed in intensive care. A few days later I had more prob-lems with my heart; this time it was a condition called atrial fibrillation. My heartbeat suddenly shot up to 190 beats per minute; it was the first time I was really afraid because my heart was pounding so hard it felt like it was coming out of my chest. But the nurse who was on duty calmed me down; I was given some medication and my heartbeat returned to normal in a matter of minutes. (Both bradycardia and atrial fibrillation are varia-tions of a general term called "heart arrhythmia," which the media often used to describe my condition.) While at St. Luke's I had at least one more episode of atrial fibrillation, which Collins later theorized had been caused by one of the chemotherapy drugs I was taking.

From May 1 to June 2 I underwent radiation therapy—high doses of therapeutic X-rays designed to kill any residual cells from the tumor in my arm—five days a week at St. Al's. Around June 7 I returned to Seattle to begin the stem-cell transplant procedure, along with my chemotherapy treatment, on an outpatient basis from the home of my sister and her hus-band in nearby Bellevue. But things didn't go smoothly. I had a sore un-derneath my arm from the radiation and I developed a tooth infection, so it was decided to extract the tooth to allow the infection to clear up, which put the whole process nearly two weeks behind schedule. I was already champing at the bit by the time the transplant regimen began on June 18. Then things really got scary.

On July 1 I was hospitalized at the Hutchinson Center because of complications stemming from the chemotherapy drugs given prior to the stem-cell transplant, which had caused me to slough the entire mucous membrane lining of my gastrointestinal tract. "His entire mucosal lining just came off, from his mouth down to his anus," Collins later told a writer. "So he ended up with bad mouth pain and throat pain; his colon was so upset that he had diarrhea that wouldn't quit until his body remade the mucosal lining."

My gastrointestinal problems were compounded by the fact I was tethered to my intravenous connections and couldn't get to the bathroom without assistance. It was like being on a five-foot leash; problem was, the bathroom was 15 feet away. Once I had really bad stomach problems, and the nurse who was on duty and helping me was really understanding. When I had to go, she would gather up all the tubes that were connected to me and follow me into the bathroom so I could relieve myself.

That was just the beginning of my problems. Patients undergoing a stem-cell transplant invariably contract some degree of infection and fever, and it is common for some to be "so severely infected to be almost at the point of death," Collins said, before their transplanted stem cells can take hold.

I was no exception. On Independence Day, Collins, who was in Boise, described my condition as "critical" after speaking to my doctors in Seattle. I was suffering from an infection caused by the absence of white blood cells in my body. I had a high fever, low blood pressure and a recurrence of the heart arrhythmia. My recovery was problematic because the stem cells that had been harvested from my body in the spring and transplanted back a couple of weeks earlier weren't expected to kick in for a few more days. I was given antibiotics and an anti-fungal drug called amphotericin, which my doctors administered in case it was a fungus rather than bacteria that was causing my fever. Amphotericin is "a very difficult medication to take because of the awful side effects—fevers, chills, kidney failure—but a drug that was necessary for Pokey in his situation," Collins said. I didn't realize it until later, but I almost died.

Here's the way *Oregonian* sportswriter Paul Buker later described the situation: "On the night of July 4, Allen's condition went beyond critical. Pumped full of painkillers and antibiotics, his speech slurred, he began suffering heart arrhythmias. His temperature shot up to 103 degrees. Jennie Kirschling, Allen's sister, told Allen's assistants he might not make it."

During my stay in the hospital my divorce was finalized. Jon Cox, my attorney, came up from Boise to Seattle to have me sign the papers; I was pretty incoherent and barely remember Jon being there. Barb, who now goes by Barbara Allen Callaghan, later married a Missoula attorney and is a bank vice president in Missoula. Everything has worked out for her; I'm glad it has.

Since the onset of my illness I must have received a couple thousand get-well cards, letters and packages, and many of them were sent while I was in Seattle that summer. At first I wanted to answer each one, but that became impossible. Believe me, that mail really helped and I greatly appreciate the fact people care about me. As I continue my fight in Canada in the fall of 1996 I'm still receiving plenty of mail from well-wishers. During my treatment in '95 I got many calls from friends and fellow coaches, including Notre Dame's Lou Holtz. In Seattle I had lots of friends—fellow coaches, colleagues, former teammates, ex-business partners from Boise, Portland and Canada—visit me during my illness. I think some of them showed up because they thought they might not see me again. That obviously wasn't the case, but I really appreciated their visits.

I was in a lot of pain during much of my hospital stay in Seattle, and the drugs I was given, which included morphine, produced some serious hallucinations. Looking back, I remember my mind doing some really strange things. One night I was totally disoriented. I had the sensation that my bed was not on the floor but nailed to the wall, and that I was in bed hanging on the wall in a vertical position. I remember being worried that if I leaned forward too far I would fall off the wall and land on my head. On another night when I was watching television it seemed I could turn completely away from the TV and still see the image on the screen, even though it was behind me.

But the weirdest episode occurred one night when I was really doped up. Around midnight, I got on the phone and called my sister and her husband in Bellevue, waking them up. "Mike Young stole my car!" I yelled into the phone. Young, my roommate and fellow coach, was in Boise and so was my car. But I was adamant that he had taken my vehicle. "Pokey, you must be hallucinating," Jennie said reassuringly. "Go back to bed."

An hour or so later, I called Jennie and Jack again. "Mike stole my car!" I yelled. "Get my car back for me!"

"Pokey," Jennie said, not quite so soothingly this time. "It's 2 o'clock in the morning. Mike is in Boise. Your car is in Boise. You're in Seattle. Go back to sleep."

I called a third time, again insisting that Mike had stolen my car and demanding that Jennie and Jack do something about it. When I called the fourth time at around 4 a.m., Jack answered. "Pokey, we found your car," he said. "Don't worry about it. Mike brought it back. Now go to bed."

"Oh, OK," I said. "Great. Thanks. Goodnight."

My condition eventually stabilized, and I returned to my sister's home on July 16. But on July 20 I was readmitted to the Hutchinson Center because of another fever. "I think that was his hardest hospitalization," Collins later said. "He was depressed and starting to wonder if he was ever going to get back to Boise."

She was right. My treatment was behind schedule; I was back in the hospital plagued by diarrhea, infections and exhaustion; I was sick, unhappy and miserable; and my August 1 deadline was in serious jeopardy. I thought I should have been well by then but I wasn't; my treatment in Seattle had become a monumental struggle physically and emotionally.

From the outset of my treatment, my objective was to be back in Boise and on the job by August 1—cancer or no cancer. After all, the whole reason I decided to undergo the stem-cell transplant was because I assumed I'd be done with it and ready to coach by the time our summer practice sessions rolled around in mid-August, which was now just three weeks away. I must admit, if BSU hadn't been rated No. 1 in the nation in some publications or if we hadn't enjoyed the kind of season we did the year before, I might not have been as anxious to return so quickly.

"He definitely had a deadline," Collins later told a reporter. "Despite his physical problems, he was pushing to get out of Seattle as soon as he could. He was going to get back to Boise. He was going to be back in the summer, and he was going to be on the football field when practice started. Period." To my frustration, however, my doctors in Seattle were not working within the same time frame. In their opinion, I was still too weak to leave, a diagnosis that did not surprise Collins. "It's not uncommon for people to go to Seattle for a stem-cell transplant and stay for three months or a hundred days," she said.

I was very despondent, and my sister and her husband were also growing concerned about my sagging spirits; in their opinion, this wasn't just a minor bout of depression. "I talked to Jennie every day on the phone," Collins recalled. "She told me more than once, 'Carolyn, we've got to get him home. He's going to die if we leave him here. He has to go home.'"

Fortunately, Collins knew the physicians in Seattle; she also had come to understand what makes me tick. In addition to her in-depth knowledge of my physical condition, Collins had also developed an understanding of my psyche—and my absolute need to coach football. Collins, who had joined St. Al's in 1994 after serving 10 years as an assistant professor in medical oncology and orthopedics at the University of Washington's medical school, interceded on my behalf. "I suspect part of the reason his doctors allowed him to come home when they did was because they knew me," she said later.

Finally, on July 27, I returned to Boise. My brother-in-law Jack, an insurance executive, made arrangements with Boise businessmen and BSU boosters Jon Miller and Allen Noble, who paid for a chartered plane that allowed a hospital-to-hospital transfer from the Hutchinson Center to St. Alphonsus. I was still so sick, I hardly remember the flight. After a brief stay at St. Al's, I was released. "But he was a mess," Collins said. "He had lost a lot of weight. He looked terrible and he felt terrible."

NONETHELESS, I MET my goal: I was back in Boise. "Pokey was bound and determined to be back here by August 1, and I'll be damned if he didn't do it with a day to spare," Max Corbet, BSU's senior sports information director, told a reporter. "I remember him walking through the [Varsity Center] doors on July 31."

But my ordeal had taken its toll. My seven-month battle with cancer had left me gaunt and emaciated; I had dropped more than 40 pounds. "It was shocking how frail he looked when he first got back," Corbet recalled. "It was like if you blew at him too hard, he might fall over."

During the first few weeks of August I had to make periodic visits to St. Al's for treatment, but when the Broncos started their summer practice sessions on August 15 I was there to welcome the players. And as the 1995 football season approached, my face became more prominent on local television sports shows; I was told later that people who had not seen me on TV since the previous winter were aghast at my appearance. I had no hair on my head, no color in my face and no meat on my bones. I was described as haggard and hollow-eyed, and I felt as bad as I looked.

During the beginning of double days Mason kept telling me, "Pokey, we can take care of practice. Why don't you just go rest? It's OK, really; we'll take care of it." But after what I had been through, I was more determined than ever to be out there on the field with the team. "No," I told Mason. "This is where I belong; this is where I want to be."

My spirit was willing but my body was a wreck; our two-a-day practices were exhausting. "Allen is frail and prone to doze off in his office chair," wrote the *Oregonian's* Paul Buker, who visited me during those summer drills, "but considering everything—considering the fact he wasn't even supposed to be alive after what happened on July 4—he's in pretty decent shape."

"The situation he was in, you wouldn't wish that on anybody," wideout Ryan Ikebe told Buker. "For him to come through it and be here for two-a-days is pretty remarkable. I thought he'd show up for a couple of hours a day, but he stays all practice long, both practices."

Another media representative who chronicled my return to the BSU football program that summer was Scott Howard-Cooper of the *Los Angeles Times*. A few years earlier Howard-Cooper had written a lighthearted story about our zany promotions and gridiron successes at Portland State. This time around, the tone of his article was not so humorous.

"He can handle the cancer and the chemotherapy and the radiation and the baldness and the gaunt look and the constant exhaustion and the realization that it was fourth-and-long for a while. ... But Pokey Allen has reached his limit," Howard-Cooper wrote. "The Boise State football team's new season is barely 26 hours old, just the second morning of two-a-days, and already practice has become sloppy, unenthusiastic. ... As if Allen would trade the moment. Eight months after a grapefruit-sized growth was found on his right triceps, about five months after surgery removed the tumor and part of the muscle, seven weeks after he almost died in a Seattle hospital from the side effects of chemotherapy and a cell transplant, and three weeks after admitting to himself he couldn't make the start of practice, he has done just that. 'I don't think he wants it to motivate us,' quarterback Tony Hilde said, 'but I think that is what's going to happen.' In return, the Broncos, a favorite for the Division I-AA title, may reward Allen with his first national championship after a couple of second-place finishes at Portland State and another at Boise State in 1994. Eighteen starters are back from that 13-2 team. And so is the coach."

Yes, I was back, but it was a struggle. "I remember walking into his office in August a couple of times between the team's double sessions and Pokey would be lying there on his couch trying to rest," recalled sportscaster Paul J. Schneider, who does BSU's radio play-by-play. "He would just be out of it, a total wreck. Yet he would get up and do the interview every time. I honestly don't know how he did it. He looked absolutely terrible."

Despite my weakened condition, I tried to make light of my situation as I described my lifestyle changes to the *Oregonian's* Buker in his article: "Allen says the cancer has been such a nuisance, his annual trip to Flathead Lake in Montana was a scratch," Buker wrote. "And his favorite Boise bar, Piper's Pub, might as well be boarded shut. 'I went there two weeks ago and had two cranberry juice and sodas,' Allen said. "I used to be big there, but bars aren't as much fun if you can't drink.'

"Allen rubs his bald head again. 'What an awful summer. No beer. No barbecues. No golf. No sex.' ... This is one life-and-death struggle that won't be on *Oprah*, Allen promises, although the media seem intent on turning him into some kind of medical breakthrough. 'I'm not doing any more treatments,' Allen said, cringing at the memory of what months of intense chemotherapy did to his body. 'If the cancer comes back, I'll just grab hold of my butt and kiss it goodbye.'"

Chapter 14

Fighting Back

With 18 starters coming back from the team that played for the Division I-AA championship the previous December, it's no wonder at least three national publications had Boise State listed as their No. 1 preseason pick in 1995. Our passing combo of quarterback Tony Hilde and wide receiver Ryan Ikebe and our entire offensive line were back, as were All-America cornerback Rashid Gayle and seven other defensive first stringers. Unfortunately, our other returning All-American, running back K.C. Adams, was an academic casualty and left the program. Even so, we looked loaded—at least on paper. But for some reason, something was missing from our 1995 squad. Actually it was several things.

First of all, Al Borges was gone. My longtime offensive coordinator had left the program following the 1994 season to take the same position with the University of Oregon. Borges, who took running back coach Tom Osborne to Eugene with him, hesitated when he was initially offered the job because he didn't want to appear to be deserting me on my sickbed. But I told Al not to concern himself with my illness and that he should take the job. I think Borges eventually wants to coach in the NFL, and I didn't think he could accomplish that by staying with me. By joining a Pac-10 school his chances of advancing to the pros are much better. And the more prestigious the school the better the chances; I'm certain that's why he moved on to UCLA after one year with the Ducks.

Following Borges' departure I named defensive coordinator Tom Mason as assistant head coach and promoted offensive line coach Dave Stromswold to offensive coordinator. I also hired Scott Criner, an assistant at BSU from 1981 to 1984, as our running back coach and former Portland State player and assistant Andy Ludwig as our QB coach. Holdovers Barry Sacks, Ron Gould, Pete Kwiatkowski and Don Bailey rounded out our coaching staff.

Despite the loss of Borges we still had an outstanding staff, and we clearly had the players necessary to make another run at the Division I-AA title, which, incidentally, would be BSU's last shot at a national crown (for a few years, anyway) since we were scheduled to join the Division I-A Big West the following season.

But something else was missing. There's no question that our success the previous year was due in large part to the leadership of seniors on that team—Joe O'Brien, Jarett Hausske, Chris Cook and Stephan Reid—guys who weren't afraid to step up and lead by word and example. Sure, we replaced them with new bodies in the lineup, but the leadership—the character—that they provided was what made the difference in '94. We had 24 seniors on that '95 squad, but with the exception of linebacker Brian Smith, nobody seemed to want to step forward and assume the leader's mantle.

Sometimes an individual or a team can amass an impressive number of victories with nothing but talent. To win it all, however, most champions must be not only talented, but also tough. Take Michael Jordan. Sure, his skills are unparalleled, but what makes him the best basketball player—and his team the best basketball team—is his undying desire to win. Our 1994 team had a small but inspirational group of leaders whose personalities and enormous spirit seemed to push the younger players beyond everyone's expectations—right to the national championship game. And that group included Tony Hilde. It's always important to have a hard-nosed quarterback. I think that's the most important position for toughness. If the quarterback isn't tenacious, then the rest of the team has trouble being tough. But Hilde had a lot of problems in 1995; all the adverse publicity he received in the *Idaho Statesman* that summer and fall didn't allow him to be as tough—to be the leader that he should have been.

We weren't as hungry in 1995 either. I think it's human nature to relax and rest on your laurels after a championship season, and that's what happened to us. We weren't really ready to play at the same level as we had the previous season. We had a lot of people who thought we were destined to be national champions that year. They read too many press clippings that said the '95 squad would be one of the best teams in BSU history, but it wasn't. We weren't as good as the year before. The 1994 team fought hard and pulled off miraculous wins. People don't realize how difficult and draining it is to win games like that week after week for an entire season. You've got to have some character and some tough kids. Although many of the same athletes played in both '94 and '95, it was like two different teams. The '95 team wasn't as tough and didn't care as much.

In retrospect, however, I know the main problem in '95 was me; I simply came back from my cancer treatment too soon. Our football team had come off an incredible season, and I just didn't want to miss out on what many originally thought would be another banner year at BSU. Looking back, it was a stupid decision. Not only for me, but I think it would have helped the team to have a healthy coach. I could see that some of our players had gotten pretty big heads after our 13-2 campaign and all the preseason hype in '95. I think under normal circumstances I could have nipped that attitude in the bud, but I didn't have the energy to do anything about it.

I can remember the first time I addressed the entire team at the start of double days. I thought I would be healthier than I was. But I was still extremely ill and exhausted from my seven-month battle with cancer. As I talked to the players, I remember my legs were shaking because I felt so weak; I barely had enough strength to finish my speech. That's when I knew—when I had some doubts as to whether I was doing the right thing.

THEN CAME OUR problems with the *Idaho Statesman*. It all began when we were recruiting running back Calvin Branch, a transfer from Iowa State whose background, we found out later, wasn't squeaky clean. Before I went to Seattle in June to undergo my stem-cell transplant and other cancer treatments, Jim Walden, Branch's coach at Iowa State, called and said Branch wanted to transfer to another school because he, Walden, was no longer the Cyclones' coach. Walden said Branch was a great kid and an outstanding running back; I don't recall anything being said about any legal problems. So we decided to talk to Branch, who was also being recruited by Colorado State and Washington State.

I had been in Boise about a week following my hospital-to-hospital transfer and was making one of my periodic visits to St. Al's in early August when Tom Mason called. He said that *Statesman* sportswriter Mike Prater was pursuing a story that said Branch had been in trouble with the law, which led to the loss of his scholarship at ISU and a three-game suspension by Dan McCarney, Walden's replacement. Mason knew about a parking-pass problem, which turned out to be a guilty plea to a misdemeanor theft charge involving the possession of a fake university parking permit. The *Statesman's* front-page story also reported that Branch, who eventually selected CSU and had a standout career with the Rams, had pleaded guilty to one count of check forgery in 1994. "He served his sentence, as far as I'm concerned ... he deserves another shot," Mason said in the article.

I agreed. "This kid is worth the risk," I told the *Statesman* in a follow-up article, adding that we had decided not to pursue five other potential recruits during the off-season because of various background problems. I will admit we should have done our homework better, and I don't mean to gloss over Branch's lawbreaking. But his parking-permit violation resulted in a $60 fine and the check he forged was for $29. Did he break the law? Definitely. Was it newsworthy? Sure. Front-page news? Well, I know it's a newspaper's responsibility to gather the news and present that information as it sees fit, but I think it was overkill.

Then came Hilde's problems, starting with the Camel's Back Park incident. In the early morning hours of August 27 he scuffled with Boise police officers who confronted him for being in a park after dark, a violation of city law. Hilde, who had been at a party with some friends following a team scrimmage earlier that evening, tried to flee from the officers, was caught, put up a struggle, and was arrested and charged with battery of a police officer, assault on an officer, resisting arrest, and being in a city park after dark—all misdemeanors. All but one of the charges were eventually dismissed and he was sentenced to 100 hours of community service the following spring and placed on unsupervised probation for a single assault charge. I don't know all the circumstances behind what happened that night, and I'm not making excuses for Hilde; he was obviously in the wrong place at the wrong time and used extremely poor judgment by running from the police. I also can't argue with the *Statesman's* front-page coverage of the incident in the ensuing days; it's definitely news when the star quarterback of the local college football team gets arrested.

Certainly, the charges against Hilde were "pretty serious," I told the *Statesman* the day after the incident. "But from what I understand it's a misdemeanor and if it's a misdemeanor, how serious can it be? He's never done anything wrong in his life. I'm a firm believer in your track record. If you're in trouble a lot, there's a point where it's the end of the line. But for somebody with no problems, and Tony has never caused any problems, you view that with a different deal." After speaking to Hilde later that day and gathering what information I had, I placed him on probation for drinking beer, a violation of team rules, but did not suspend him. The primary reason for my decision, I reiterated at a press conference on August 28, was because Hilde had no previous problems with the law, which, it turned out, wasn't totally accurate and came to light three days later in the *Statesman*.

A month earlier Hilde had been in a car accident in Washington state. He and a companion told Washington Patrol officers that Tony was the passenger, but they later admitted Hilde was behind the wheel when the accident occurred. On August 31 the *Statesman* broke the story with a front-page article by Prater which reported that Hilde had been charged with obstruction of justice—a charge that was later dropped. When I took no further disciplinary action against Hilde, I came under fire the next day in the *Statesman*.

In addition to another Page One story that reported my response to the new charges against Hilde, the paper torched me on its editorial page— I guess a similar editorial that criticized me two days earlier wasn't quite enough—with a piece that highlighted a quote from a statement I had made earlier in the week: "'I have trouble getting real excited about misdemeanors.'—BSU football coach Pokey Allen," the quote read. The editorial went on to say, "If Allen can't get excited about misdemeanors, then how about respect for the law? Character? Responsibility? Lying? Leadership? … Allen downplayed accusations that Hilde [scuffled with police] at a Boise park. Allen also assured the public that Hilde's background was clean. Yet, two days later, Allen said he was aware of additional charges against Hilde in the state of Washington. …"

OK, I was vaguely aware that Hilde was in a traffic accident, which occurred the day after I returned to Boise in a hospital-to-hospital airplane transfer from Seattle to St. Alphonsus Regional Medical Center. When I returned to the BSU football offices a few days later, Mason told me about Hilde's accident and that it "had been taken care of" and that I shouldn't worry about it. At the August 28 press conference I did erroneously state that Hilde had no previous problems with the law before because I assumed, incorrectly, that his traffic accident was not an issue.

Would I have done some things differently? Perhaps. Was I too lenient with Hilde? I don't think so. The fact of the matter is this: When I returned to Boise in late July I was incoherent the first few days and still quite ill from the side effects of the extensive chemotherapy, stem-cell transplant and associated treatments that I had undergone at the Hutchinson Center. I hardly remember the plane trip from Seattle to Boise or being admitted to St. Al's; in the ensuing days I was working in the office for a few hours and spending nights in the hospital, trying to regain my strength and overcome the constant exhaustion and sickness that had racked my body. So when I was told Hilde's mishap wasn't a problem, I left it at that. With all my infirmities at that time, some people say I shouldn't have been coaching, and in hindsight they were probably right, but I think the *Statesman* could have cut me some slack back then.

Unfortunately, Hilde's legal problems didn't end with the 1995 season. In February 1996 his name once again appeared on the front page of the *Statesman* in regard to a stolen campus parking pass that was found in his vehicle. Fed up with it all, Hilde, who had one year of eligibility remaining, announced that he would not participate in spring football drills because of the effect the bad publicity was having on the team, and that his future with the BSU football program was "up in the air." He was fined $25 for using a stolen parking permit, which he and roommate and teammate Ryan Ikebe claimed belonged to Ikebe. Ikebe said he purchased the permit from an unidentified student who said he was leaving school. Hilde remained in school for the spring 1996 semester and decided to return to the program in the fall for his senior season.

What about the statement about not getting excited about misdemeanors? It was taken out of context and part of a lengthy interview with Prater that I *thought* was off the record (although I made a similar comment during the August 28 press conference). My intent was to say something like this: Given everything I had been through—a life-threatening illness, utter exhaustion and a couple of brushes with death in the preceding months—I had trouble getting real excited about misdemeanors as opposed to more serious crimes. I admit the actual quote wasn't the smartest thing I ever said, but I thought Prater knew me well enough to grasp the meaning of my words and not misinterpret them.

It was under those adverse circumstances that we opened the 1995 season on September 9 against Utah State and first-year coach John L. Smith in Logan. Despite my weakened condition, I was at my accustomed spot on the sidelines. "We were all watching Pokey as he stepped out onto the field for the pregame warm-ups at Romney Stadium that night," said Paul J. Schneider, BSU's play-by-play radio announcer in an interview. "He still looked bad, but he kind of had this satisfied look on his face. It was like he was saying, 'Yeah, I did it. I made it.' At that moment, Pokey set a standard for personal courage that I have never seen before in my life."

Mason agreed: "I don't think many of us could have done what he did that night. I still remember, it was a nice, warm evening, but he was really sick and shivering on the sidelines. We put sweaters on him, and he was still shivering. But he was out there coaching his team; he was sicker than hell but he wasn't going to be denied. It was like he was saying, 'I'll be damned if someone's gonna say I can't coach this team.' I'll tell you, he's one tough son of a bitch."

Hilde and Ikebe hooked up for a 77-yard TD pass, Andre Horace returned a kickoff 94 yards for another score, and Greg Erickson kicked a 21-yard field goal as we took a 17-6 lead at halftime over the Aggies. Then our offensive line took control of the game in the second half as Hilde engineered three more scoring drives en route to a 38-14 win. Interestingly, it was our second victory in as many games against Smith, who was the head coach at Idaho the previous season. After being tormented by Smith's outstanding UI teams from 1989 through 1993, I'm sure there were a lot of Bronco fans who took pleasure in beating him twice in a row.

After that game, I considered taking a medical leave of absence for the remainder of the season because I thought I was too sick to do my job. But after what had happened to Hilde and all the bad publicity we were getting in the *Statesman*, I thought it might appear as if I was stepping down under fire. If it hadn't been for the *Statesman*, I probably would have taken some time off—perhaps the rest of the season—to recuperate. Looking back, I probably should have done it for the players and assistant coaches; not for me, but because it wasn't fair to them. It was a difficult and demanding job for the condition I was in. If the head coach can't do his job, then the assistant coaches can't do their jobs either. If I had taken a leave of absence, Tom Mason would have been fine as acting head coach. There would have been no problem.

THROUGHOUT MY CAREER I've dealt with members of the press in the same manner I do most other people. I have found only a small number of media representatives to be intrusive and unfair, and in both Portland and Boise I think I am well-liked by the local media because I am open and obliging—to a fault in the opinion of some of my coaching colleagues and sports information directors. Cripes, I allowed Carolyn Holly of Boise TV station KTVB to be on hand when I had my tumor surgically removed the previous March. If *that's* not being cooperative with the press, I don't know what is.

I know I come up with my share of predictable and trite comments during interviews and press conferences, but I also know that over the years I have provided my share of good "copy" and column fodder for reporters and journalists. My popularity with the media was never the result of some insincere scheme to polish my image or enhance my standing in the community; I simply believe that good rapport with the press makes everybody's job easier, and it's a rare occasion when I don't grant an interview, even when it's an inconvenience.

In fact, at Portland State I think part of the reason we received such good coverage was that we almost always cooperated with the media. By doing that, I think the members of the Portland press got to know—and like—our football team and our people better than they knew the Oregon and Oregon State football teams. Often, one of the Portland TV sports guys would come up to me in the middle of practice and say his station didn't have anything good for the sports segment of the evening news and ask if he could get a quick quote from a player. I figured, hey, this is football; it isn't some secretive thing, and I would pull a player out of practice and let the sportscaster do the interview. I mean, it only took or minute or two. What's the big deal?

In my first two seasons at BSU my relationship with the *Idaho States-man* was congenial, and in general I thought the paper's coverage of our football program—from the tough times of 1993 through the euphoria of '94—was balanced and accurate. Moreover, after I was diagnosed with cancer in December 1994, I thought the paper chronicled the first seven months of my ordeal in an empathetic and unobtrusive manner. I'm also grateful for the many kind words and supportive editorials that have appeared on the *Statesman's* opinion page in regard to my battle with the disease.

The 1995 season was another story, however. The adverse publicity the BSU football program received in the *Statesman* in the late summer and fall of that year was a nightmare. I don't deny that certain off-the-field incidents merited the media coverage they received, nor do I dispute any of the basic facts the paper reported in regard to transgressions committed by some BSU football players and recruits. Nor do I take such wrongdoing lightly—despite the *Statesman's* inference to the contrary.

I take offense at certain articles written during that time for three reasons: First is the way some of those "facts" were presented to exaggerate the seriousness and scope of certain misdeeds by BSU football players and recruits; second is the "play" some of those uncomplimentary stories received in the paper; and third is what I perceived as a "gotcha" journalism mentality at the *Statesman* as our program's problems mounted.

The days when the *Statesman* was hammering on me, the program in general, and Tony Hilde in particular were very tough times. Should the *Statesman* have ignored or downplayed the problems Hilde and other players had with the law? Of course not. But in my opinion the paper went out of its way to find dirt on BSU football players—information that at times was old and innocuous—and then blew it out of proportion.

Again, I don't mean to minimize violations of the law, but if you have around 100 college-aged kids running around, you're bound to find some unacceptable conduct—and the *Statesman* certainly did as it launched an investigation into any and all unlawful behavior by players in our program. The low point came on September 14, five days after our season-opening win at Utah State. Going back to 1992, the newspaper detailed scrapes with the law by 15 BSU football players and two walk-ons who left the team before the season began. The same front-page article also noted that I had suspended reserve fullback John Tia, who two nights earlier had been arrested and charged with two misdemeanors after he got into a tussle with an Ada County sheriff's deputy outside a campus study hall. The *Statesman* also considered it necessary to print mug shots of the 17 BSU football players named in the report, listing their offenses—all of them misdemeanors that ranged from battery to driving while under the influence.

But that wasn't the worst of it. In an accompanying article the *Statesman* reported that Boise State had "misreported the criminal troubles of its athletes" to the state. The paper's charge was in reference to the school's response to a request by the State Board of Education for BSU and Idaho's other two universities to submit reports about legal troubles of student-athletes following a series of offenses by Idaho State football players. Based on a check with the school's coaches, university officials originally reported seven incidents over the previous 12 months in which BSU student-athletes had brushes with the law. The university did not check local court records or talk to police in preparing its report, as the *Statesman* decided to do. The paper also arbitrarily decided to go back three years in coming up with its numbers. The university amended the report to 17, but the damage had been done. In the wake of the *Statesman's* report, BSU president Charles Ruch announced a "zero tolerance" policy stating that any student-athlete who ran afoul of the law would face immediate punishment.

To be sure, you can't ignore violations of the law and criminal behavior. But in my opinion the *Statesman* sought to distort the information it had and portray the BSU football program in the worst possible light. Why? I have no idea. I thought the whole thing was a terrible injustice to somebody like Brian Smith. I mean, here was a kid from the mean streets of Tacoma who had some problems in the past but had stayed out of trouble for a year and a half, kept his nose clean, worked hard toward a degree, and had emerged as a leader on our team; now all of a sudden his past indiscretions are trotted out for the whole world to see.

Then John Costa, the *Statesman's* executive editor, followed up with a column a week and a half later that ripped the university's administration, saying it had "submitted a flawed effort" in its report to the state board. In the column, Costa, whom I have never met, said he had been asked why the paper found it necessary to publish names, pictures and arrest details of the players. "This caused as much pain as anything we did," he wrote, "but I firmly believe that not giving precise detail is worse than giving it. If we didn't name the players, the whole team becomes suspect. ... So, once we named them, I thought we had to describe the offenses, because they vary in severity. This story is very painful."

Gee ... how touching. But Costa never did explain why the photos of the players were published—even though he posed the question himself in his column. And I thought his "flawed effort" comment was also unfair. The state board gave no specific instructions when it asked BSU, ISU and the University of Idaho to submit reports on legal troubles of student-athletes, and I don't think it was expecting the schools to run the names of their athletes through county court records. Just like UI and ISU, Boise State submitted its original—and admittedly lower—number of charges against student-athletes based on a good-faith effort.

I suppose some people might think BSU's initial report *was* incomplete, but in my opinion, the *Statesman* went out of its way to come up with the largest number of student-athlete offenses it could find. As mentioned, two of the 17 players listed were walk-ons who had quit the team *before the season even started*, and two others were cited for underage drinking *while they were in high school*. What do those misdeeds have to do with the BSU football program? Well, I don't know. And while the *Statesman* decided to print names, pictures and arrest details, it failed to mention how the players pleaded to the charges. Some of the charges were pending at the time and some of the players pleaded not guilty, but I guess that would have lessened the impact of the paper's story. At the risk of sounding like I don't take lawbreaking seriously, I should point out that most of the offenses were for illegal consumption of alcohol, which most young people do at one time or another.

Costa also noted that "the third-string fullback [Tia] was booted from the team for one known misdemeanor charge [while] the starting quarterback [Hilde] is still playing with two. ... The royalty of the Bronco football team," he wrote, "is spared the fate of the commoners."

First of all, Tia was suspended, not "booted" from the team. Second, the team rules had changed following Hilde's run-in with the police; Tia's scuffle took place after our players were told that any further incidents would not be tolerated and thus would be dealt with severely. If Tia had committed his transgression first, his punishment would have been the same as Hilde's; had Hilde been the second to run afoul of the law, he would have received the same penalty Tia did. Third, Costa's accusation of a double standard between star and backup players was also false. Earlier that season—before his column was published—I had already suspended defensive tackle Sione Fifita, perhaps the best player on the team, and defensive back Kevin Chiles, a key reserve, because of criminal charges.

I don't dispute the *Statesman's* right to print the news in an objective manner, and neither, I assume, does Boise attorney Raymond Schild. I've never met Schild, but someone showed me a column he wrote in the October 9, 1995, issue of the *Idaho Business Review*, which I thought made some excellent points in regard to responsible journalism.

Commenting that the media often use the First Amendment's freedom-of-speech protection "as a shield and a sword" to invade what otherwise would be the rights of individuals, Schild wrote: "Pokey Allen, having fought a herculean battle with cancer, having suffered, strived and, God willing, defeated such an awesome foe, has done so at the expense of a great deal of his emotional and physical energy.

"Is it responsible to put such a man through the wringer, questioning every decision that is made as to whether Athlete A or Athlete B will or will not be suspended because of alleged criminal or other wrongdoing? Since when did the school and the coach become responsible for the private lives of [their] athletes?

"Since when did BSU become a particular target? … Does anyone still seriously believe that every athlete is to be held to the standard of a role model and have every action and activity scrutinized against a standard of perfection? … Unfettered [First Amendment] protection, or nearly so, provides incentives for and induces trampling on the rights of others."

Yes, the actions of some of our football players were an embarrassment to our program and the university. Yes, some of the 17 charged players broke the law. Yes, in some cases their actions merited coverage in the paper. But in the overbearing manner in which it was done by the *Statesman* in 1995? I don't think so.

And neither does Boise sportswriter Art Lawler, who happened to be the *Statesman's* sports editor at the time. In 1996 Lawler left the *Statesman* and began a publication titled *BroncoFaxtra*, a four-times-a-week online newsletter that covers BSU sports. In the November 2, 1996, edition of his publication, Lawler provided his perspective of the *Statesman's* coverage of the BSU football team's legal problems the previous year. Lawler said he hadn't previously written on the subject for two reasons: First, he feared anything he wrote would come across like an it-wasn't-my-fault self-exoneration; second, he worried about being labeled as "an apologist for the unlawful behavior of Boise State athletes," neither of which do I consider to be the case.

Some excerpts: "Those [BSU] stories went to the front page from day one … they were orchestrated by editors much higher up the ladder than me. ... But I did have my opinions ... I just wasn't allowed to express them. I was overruled, not once, but several times. ... When Tony Hilde had his problems with law-enforcement officials, the stories all landed on the front page, and I don't think all of them were front-page news. I also think the so-called 'wanted' poster pictures of other Broncos involved in misdemeanors was overkill. At best they were discriminatory.

"To bring in the minor-in-possession-of-alcohol offenses of kids, some of which went as far back as high school, I think was inappropriate. It reaches the point of seeing how bad a paper can make a football team look. It has the appearance of 'How many players—even if they're no longer on campus—can you add to get the misdemeanor total up?' Nobody ever said that, it just looks that way."

Regarding my comments about not caring about misdemeanors, Lawler wrote: "I know Pokey Allen, and to suggest that he doesn't take lawbreaking activities of his players seriously is to greatly judge and underestimate the man as an ethical human being. If you know Pokey, you know he gave stern warnings to his players about such things. ... Here's a guy who's been on all kinds of medication, who's just fought his way back from death with the stem-cell transplant, and you're taking him down because he's not explaining himself effectively."

With all the crap our team was taking from the *Statesman*, it's no wonder our players decided not to speak to Prater after the paper printed the 17 "wanted" poster shots. The *Statesman's* repeated negative stories were, to the players, unfair, so why cooperate with him? I didn't instruct them to give Prater the cold shoulder; when they broached the subject with me, I told them I would support whatever they decided. It was the players' idea originally, and as far as I'm concerned, they should have stuck with it.

As for me? Sure I was upset by the whole thing, and given a second chance I would have chosen my words more carefully in a few instances. But I tried not to let the bad publicity bother me. The fact that I had the backing of athletic director Gene Bleymaier sure helped. Somebody in the local media called me BSU's "embattled" coach during those troublesome weeks. Hell, I was never embattled! I know president Ruch was unhappy when the *Statesman's* report came out, but neither he nor Bleymaier ever second-guessed the disciplinary action I took, and I was never called on the carpet by either of them.

DESPITE THE TURMOIL caused by the *Statesman*, we defeated Sam Houston State 38-14 in our home opener on September 16 as Hilde threw four touchdown passes and ran for another score. The following Saturday there was yet another article in the *Statesman,* this time about a ruckus, reportedly involving BSU football players, outside a Boise bar following the Sam Houston State game, though charges were never filed.

In spite of my illness and all the distractions, we had managed to win our first two contests. But I had some real misgivings about our football team. We weren't practicing or playing like a team on a mission. At the time I felt like I was stuck. I didn't have the energy to turn it around, but I didn't feel I could relinquish my coaching duties either; I wasn't about to give the *Statesman* the satisfaction that it had forced me to step down—mistaken as that notion would have been. So I stayed, knowing we were in for a rude awakening.

Montana proved me right. We went up to Missoula and got mauled by the Grizzlies 54-28 as Dave Dickenson exacted a measure of revenge from the beating he took the year before with 383 yards passing and a school-record six TD passes. (UM went on to win the Division I-AA national title that year.) Hilde, meanwhile, did not complete any of his nine passes and was forced to leave the game with an injury.

"Still, even with the defeat, it's unlikely Boise State will find itself any less popular [with local fans]," reported Samantha Stevenson of the *New York Times,* who came to Boise to write an article on our team's troubles with the *Statesman.* Observing that "the city has become more supportive of its team as additional details about the [misbehavior of] football players have been made public. ... The newspaper's disclosures seem to have united the community against the *Statesman.* ... Instead of applauding the *Statesman* for exposing problems—problems the newspaper says that Boise State shares to some extent with the national champion Nebraska Cornhuskers—many residents criticize the paper for equating youthful indiscretions with serious felony allegations."

Stevenson's mention of Nebraska was in reference to a *Statesman* article that compared our problems—and the resultant negative publicity—to a spate of crimes allegedly committed by Cornhusker student-athletes during the 1995 season. Boise State and Nebraska? I mean, come on—about the only thing the BSU and Nebraska football programs have in common is the fact they both play in their state capitals.

Anyway, after we got pasted by Montana, we lost back-to-back home games—22-17 to Northwestern State of Louisiana and 32-13 to Northern Arizona. By then it was painfully obvious we didn't have the same focus or attitude from the year before. Our players didn't perform well and our staff didn't coach very well during our three-game tailspin; I was having serious doubts about my ability to return to good health and coach effectively. "This team looks like it's a team without a very good football coach," I told the *Statesman's* Prater after our loss to the Lumberjacks on October 7. "The problem is this team doesn't have a head coach with the energy to get things done. In retrospect, I think this team would have been better off if I hadn't come back so early. I don't have the range of emotions you need to be a good head coach. I feel better if I'm a grouch and an asshole. I don't think coming back so fast was a good decision for me. ... That doesn't mean I'm gonna quit now. I guarantee you that I'm not gonna quit in the middle of the season."

"Allen's season has been one of grit and little glory, a sharp contrast to 1994 when the Broncos made it to the Division I-AA title game before losing to Youngstown State," wrote the *Oregonian's* Bob Robinson.

Finally, around the halfway point of the season, I started feeling better; ever so slowly I began to regain my strength and stamina. Correspondingly, our staff started coaching better and the players began to perform better. After those three straight losses I got actively involved. I started yelling and screaming. It takes a lot of energy to get mad, and I have found that players usually don't listen unless you get a certain tone in your voice; without that tone, you have no chance. By mid-October I finally had the strength to use my voice, be an asshole when necessary, and take control of the team again. I went out and raised hell on the practice field, and all of a sudden we were back on track. When I walked out on the practice field and quit allowing the players to loaf, and started to mete out punishment for goofing off with belly slammers and sprints, from that moment on I knew we were going to be a decent football team.

We ended our three-game losing streak with a 40-14 conference victory over Weber State in Ogden as Hilde ran 42 yards for a touchdown and threw a pair of TD passes to tight end Bernie Zimmerman. Then we beat Idaho State at home 27-17 as Rashid Gayle returned an interception 47 yards for a TD.

I'm no magician or miracle worker, but I know what works for me. People have said I have charisma, which is defined as "a personal magic or leadership arousing special popular loyalty or enthusiasm for a public figure." I don't know about that, but if I have control of a situation I like my chances. When I was captain of the University of Utah football team my senior year in college, I always thought we had a chance to win when I was at quarterback. The same goes for when I played quarterback in high school. As an athlete, if you exhibit leadership qualities, if you are unselfish and know how to motivate your teammates, you can often find a way to win. It's basically the same way with coaching.

"Boise State quarterback Tony Hilde noticed the difference in his coach two weeks ago," the *Oregonian's* Robinson wrote the week after the ISU win. "The subdued Pokey Allen of early in the season suddenly began to act a little more like the Pokey Allen of old. 'He started bringing a new intensity to practice,' Hilde said. 'He hadn't been very vocal early in the season, but now he is more a part of our day-to-day stuff again. It was infectious to the players. I think it had a lot to do with the way we've played in the last two weeks.'"

We beat Portland State 49-14 as Hilde threw three touchdown passes, two to Ikebe. The next week we outscored Eastern Washington 63-44. Hilde threw five TD passes and we amassed a single-game school record of 664 yards total offense. Our faint hopes for a return to the Division I-AA playoffs were revived after we posted our fifth straight win and improved to 7-3 with a 35-7 triumph over Montana State. But for any chance at a postseason berth, we knew we had to beat Idaho in Moscow in our regular-season finale.

Throughout my head coaching career, I've tried to let the players and assistants try to work things out if there are problems; I try to stay out as long as I can before I step in. I want to see how the assistant coaches and the players are going to handle it. But when I think it's time to step in, I won't hesitate. I want to make sure that we're on the right track. The 1995 season was the weirdest year I ever experienced as a head coach because until midseason I had lost my feeling for when to step in. I thought we were ready for Idaho, but I was wrong. We stayed close and trailed only 10-3 at halftime, but the playoff-bound Vandals took control in the second half and went on to win 33-13; it was the final Big Sky game for both schools.

This may sound strange, but I think our 13-2 season in 1994 was a bad thing for the respective careers of our coaches, my own career included. If we had gone 6-5, 7-4 or 8-3 our second year, most BSU fans would have considered that a significant improvement from our 3-8 record of '93, and nobody would have been unhappy with our 7-4 record in 1995. But when we had our breakout year in '94, we set ourselves up for all kinds of expectations. Everyone assumed we had turned the corner after '94, but that wasn't the case.

We gambled and went the quick fix route with an infusion of junior college transfers in hopes of having two exceptional seasons with players who would be with us for only two years. As it turned out, we only got one of the two seasons we had hoped for. The way the 1995 season turned out was really unfortunate because I think we could have built on the '94 season and created an aura of success that would be unparalleled. But my illness and all the other problems threw a monkey wrench into those plans, and we're still trying to recover.

Chapter 15

The Ultimate Challenge

T he year 1996 started well. Through the winter and into the spring the periodic CAT scans and other tests to determine if the cancer had returned were negative. My hair, such as it is, grew back and I regained much of the weight and stamina I had lost during my ordeal the previous year. By the time spring football arrived in April I had returned to my daily routine. Aside from the specter of cancer, I had no problems. "Right now I feel great, and I'm feeling better every day," I stated in an article in *FOCUS*, Boise State's alumni magazine. "But am I cancer-free? I don't think it's to that point yet. I think after two or three years they kind of declare that you have no more chance than anyone else of getting this kind of cancer, but I think there's still some doubt whether it's going to come back or not."

Like I told everyone since the start of my illness, I was not going to brood over my fate. I had weathered the harrowing experience of tumor surgery, chemotherapy, radiation and a stem-cell transplant through 1995; now I was ready to enjoy life again. And one of the first things on my list was to break out the golf clubs. Golf has become my favorite pastime over the years, and it was an exhilarating feeling to be back on the links with my friends. I also enjoyed a memorable experience in the early summer when I got to carry the Olympic torch as it came through Boise en route to the Atlanta Games. My run covered only a few hundred yards, thank God, because I still wasn't in the best of shape.

I've often been asked if I have changed since my illness. The answer is yes. I think I'm a better person and maybe a tougher person for having been through it all. And if things don't work out, I have no regrets. I'm glad I have lived my life the way I have because I haven't wasted any time. I've had fun, I've laughed. It's all been great. I still live life hard, still live for the moment. Cancer hasn't changed my attitude toward life—or the hereafter.

I know there are thousands of stories about people who undergo some sort of religious epiphany after having a brush with death or learning they have a life-threatening disease, but that hasn't happened to me. I believe there is a God, but I don't care for organized religions. I have a theory that if I live my life in an upright manner and try not to hurt other people and be honest and a stand-up kind of guy, good things are going to happen to me when it's time to cash in my chips, so to speak. I hope there is an afterlife, and if there's a place where they send good people, I think I'll deserve to be there when my time is up.

I look at it this way: There are thousands of religions in the world, all of which say their followers must live their lives a certain way or they're doomed. Well, then, that means all those millions of people who don't belong to the right religion—whichever one it is—are wrong. It doesn't make any sense to me. If God is as compassionate as everyone says He is, it seems to me He is going to take care of good people—no matter what religion they are. So I've always tried to be a good person. I hope when I go to my grave, God will look down and say, "Hey, Pokey was a good guy, he was nice to other people. Let's take care of him."

That's why one of my basic rules has always been to treat people with decency and respect. During my nearly 30 years of coaching, I hope one thing my players have learned from me is that you have to treat people well. The one thing I can't stand is a player being a jerk and treating another person badly. When one of my players gets in trouble, I'll almost always listen to his side of the story, but I have little tolerance for rude treatment of another human being. Sure, I holler at my players during practice and games, but it's not in a cruel and abusive manner like the way Bobby Knight yells. And I would never yell at a stranger—as Knight did at an event official in Boise during the NCAA basketball tournament a few years ago. I treat people like I want them to treat me. I don't yell at equipment men, at trainers or at people who would let you bully them and probably not retaliate. There's no reason to do it—and no excuse for it.

I've seen coaches who are abusive and others who act aloof and have as little interaction with players and boosters as possible. I don't agree with either of those styles; I couldn't do my job that way. I have to be close to my players and mingle and be with people. I could not have helped turn the Portland State football program around with any other personality than the one I have.

I've also been asked if I've talked to other cancer patients. I haven't sought them out, but, yes, if somebody calls and wants to talk, I'm glad to do it. One of them is Danielle Bauer of Boise. She's about six years old and she's got rhabdomyosarcoma. She can't pronounce it, so she calls it Pokey's cancer. I talk to her as often as I can and tell her that everything is going to be OK. She's the cutest little thing. She's got no hair and wears a floppy little hat. My daughter turned three in October of 1996, and I can't imagine what it would be like to have a sick child. I have also talked to some adults, and what I try to get across to them is that they're not alone and they can use me if they need me. I guess when I deal with people with diseases I'm more empathetic than I was before because now I can appreciate what they're going through.

One person who has helped me a great deal is Larry Selland, Boise State's former executive vice president who was the university's acting president when I was hired in December 1992. For the past 10 years Selland has waged his own battle against cancer with bravery and dignity. He too has sought alternative treatments for a disease that's considered incurable. He's an amazing man—a man of immense integrity. Every time we visit I come away with new insights into how to face this deadly disease. Once, when it was apparent chemotherapy wasn't going to help me, Larry sent me a computer printout that listed different hospitals throughout North America that offered alternative cancer treatments. Another time his advice was short and simple: "Just don't quit, Pokey," he said. "Don't give up. That's half the battle." Larry Selland has been through a lot more than I have. He's a great man and an inspiration.

Another question I've been asked is if my illness has put football in perspective—have I come to some realization that there are "other" things besides football? Of course. But to be honest, cancer hasn't changed my basic perspective. I still feel the same way about football that I always have. I take my job seriously; I just don't take *myself* too seriously. I've been involved in football as a player or coach for nearly 40 years, but I think I've always maintained a healthy attitude. Yes, college football is my livelihood, but it's still a game involving young people, guys who aren't full-fledged adults yet. The benefits of football? I know similar words have been expressed hundreds of times with much more eloquence, but it's a truism that football teaches about life. And for that reason I think my job is important.

Membership on any athletic team is a training ground for real life. I think football teaches plenty: competitiveness, the rewards of hard work, how to get along with other people—qualities we all need to get ahead in the "real world." The important thing about football, or any sport, is that it teaches kids how to handle success and cope with disappointment. And at the level I work, it provides many kids with a college education.

I know it's easy for people to become cynical when a coach begins to recite—as if by rote—the standard and predictable lines about maintaining the proper balance between academics and athletics, and I don't profess to have a flawless program with a perfect graduation rate. What I *can* claim, however, is a program that offers more than lip service to its student-athletes when it comes to academic support. When I first started at Boise State, I was asked in a *FOCUS* interview what I do differently in regard to academics. "I get personally involved," I replied. "No matter how many advisers you've got, how many tutors you've got, the main factor in graduating football players is that the coaches care whether they get the degree. The thing you can't do with players is bluff them. They find out pretty quick when you are just talking and not meaning it."

How do I get personally involved? At BSU we have a morning study hall called the Breakfast Club, which our coaching staff initially instituted at Portland State. Any player with a grade-point average below 2.25 is required to be part of the Breakfast Club, which runs from 7:30 to 8:30 a.m. Monday through Thursday throughout the school year. And I'm there with them. One of my assistants will occasionally sit in for me if I have a morning speaking engagement or another commitment, but I'm usually there, working with our players and showing them we're committed to their education.

I don't care if a player is a black kid from Los Angeles or a white kid from rural Idaho, I want him to come away from our program with a sense of what it is like to be a person—not a football player, but a person—and how to be part of a team and work with people of different races and social backgrounds. I've always felt that if a player has some ability, some desire and some smarts, he is going to wind up a better person for having been part of our program. We've turned out some great football players, but more important, we've turned out some great *people* both at Portland State and Boise State. That is why my job is important.

Some critics have said I take too much of a boys-will-be-boys attitude in regard to discipline, but that's nonsense; only a nitwit would insinuate something like that. I've booted players from our program when it's been warranted. But I've also refrained from taking such action when I've had a gut feeling that doing so would do more damage than good to the individual. If I allow a kid in trouble to remain with our program, we're eventually going to help him "do the right thing"; in the long run we're usually going to help him learn a few things and make him a better person. It hasn't always worked that way; I've made judgment calls that sometimes have been wrong. But to be a good football coach you have to be a good human being and show some compassion, and I'm willing to take the risk if it means giving a 20-year-old a second chance. Lord knows I needed a few breaks when I was that age.

Sure, I've given players more chances than they probably deserve on a few occasions. But if I do, and if the kid eventually comes around, I figure it was worth it because I may have played a role in helping to mold a human being who is eventually going to go out and be successful and have a positive impact on society. Trite words and overdone phrases? Perhaps. I don't claim to have the world's most expansive vocabulary. But I do know this: It has been amazing how many wrong-side-of-the-tracks kids have benefitted from being players in our program. That is why my job is important. That is why I coach. That is why I get annoyed when some members of the media who don't know the whole story about our off-the-field problems take me to task.

One person who seems to understand where I'm coming from is Art Lawler. In one of the early editions of his *BroncoFaxes*, the former *Statesman* sports editor wrote this about me: "Like all of us, [Pokey] is flawed. He likes to drink a few beers. His language could improve. He likes to date young women and have a good time. The only marriage that could ever work for Pokey is the one he has with his players and coaches. But that's a commitment never questioned."

ON JULY 1, 1996, after a 26-year affiliation with the Big Sky Conference, Boise State began a new era with its entry into the Big West Conference. In doing so our football team joined the upper echelon of the nation's collegiate programs in Division I-A.

My health continued to improve as our coaching staff prepared for BSU's inaugural season as one of the NCAA's 111 Division I-A football teams. I knew our first year in the Big West was going to be a tough one because it was going to take our program at least three years to reach the Division I-A scholarship level of 85. (The problem is that as a Division I-AA program, BSU had a cap of 63 scholarships per year, but NCAA rules prohibit schools from adding more than 25 new football scholarships per year.) Nonetheless, I was looking forward to the challenge. I actually think I'm a better coach when my staff and I are in a rebuilding or transition mode, and that certainly described our situation since we would be at an immediate disadvantage going up against opponents with the full complement of scholarships allowed to Division I-A schools.

Over the Memorial Day weekend and again in early July, I enjoyed some rest and recreation in Missoula and at my cabin at Flathead Lake. I spent some quality time with my mom, Jennie and her family and my daughter. I saw Taylor almost every evening, and my former wife Barbara brought her to see me a couple of times while I was playing golf; it was great fun chasing Taylor around the golf course. You know, I've loved my daughter since the day she was born, but I really developed an appreciation of the joys of fatherhood during that time. Those moments with her were special.

In late July I visited the Miami Dolphins training camp in Florida and attended the Big West coaches' meetings in Dallas. While at the league meetings, I was interviewed by *Forth Worth Star-Telegram* sportswriter Wendell Barnhouse about my battle with cancer. "Every six weeks Allen has a medical checkup," Barnhouse wrote in his article. "For now, rhabdomyosarcoma is just a word in [his] vocabulary, not a sinister disease."

"We had all kinds of problems on the team last year," I said in the article, "but I stopped worrying about it. When you think you could die the next day, its kind of hard to worry about whether the *Idaho Statesman* is going to write an ugly article about you." In his story Barnhouse described my fight with cancer and then asked me about my long-term prognosis. "What they know is they can't find any cancer in my body," I said. "It might be there, but so microscopic they don't know it's there. It might be back tomorrow."

Unfortunately, I was right.

I FIRST NOTICED a small lump in my chest in June, so I went to see my oncologist, Dr. Carolyn Collins. I could tell she was concerned. But when the results of the CAT scan she had ordered came back negative, I decided not to worry about it. While I was at the Big West meetings in Dallas, however, the lump seemed to have grown. Collins was on vacation when I got back to Boise, and my next CAT scan wasn't scheduled until mid-August; I didn't think I could wait. I called Collins' office at the St. Alphonsus Cancer Treatment Center and asked if someone else would do a biopsy on the lump in my chest. The biopsy was performed Monday, August 5, and the next morning I was told the growth was malignant. In addition, it was discovered that I had a small tumor on the lining of each lung. It was rhabdomyosarcoma; it had metastasized.

I was stunned. Then I was scared. Within the hour I told my boss, BSU athletic director Gene Bleymaier, and sports information director Max Corbet that the cancer was back. The contingency plan we had developed in case the cancer recurred was implemented: After Gene, Max and I met with Charles Ruch, BSU's president, I stepped down effective immediately to take a medical leave of absence and assistant head coach Tom Mason was named interim head coach.

The cruel irony to the timing of the whole thing was that August 6 was the day that summer practices were to begin for freshmen and transfers. It technically was to have been my first practice as a Division I-A head football coach. Instead, at a hastily called press conference at St. Al's, I once again had to tell the media that I had cancer. "The last time I was really positive I was going to beat it," I said. "You're not as sure the second time. I'm very nervous. I'd be lying to you if I said I wasn't. I like to act braver than I am, but I'm a little scared. I hope I stud up. I really hope I do. I'm a very optimistic person, but I remember when I went through the stem-cell transplant I think they said, 'If this doesn't work, grab hold of your rear end because you might want to kiss it goodbye.' I feel great, so it's pretty shocking. I was pretty positive I would have no problem. I really thought the test results would come back negative and everything would be OK."

But things were far from OK. Mason seemed more upset than anyone. Tom and I have been together since 1986, and we're real close. He's an outstanding person and I think he'll make a great head coach. But he obviously didn't want his first head job under these circumstances. "I'm not mentally prepared for this," he said at the press conference. "I did not think [the cancer] was going to come back."

"Tom Mason is a great coach and he is going to do a great job," I told the reporters. "I didn't want to start coaching and then stop coaching, and I didn't want to be sick while I was coaching." But I knew I had to leave the program and seek a cure right away. Otherwise I had no chance.

Nine days later, and for the second time in 17 months, Dr. Chappie Conrad performed surgery on me at the University of Washington Medical Center in Seattle in an effort to halt the spread of rhabdomyosarcoma in my body. And like the first time, the news wasn't good. Conrad and the other physicians went in and removed the tumor in my chest and on the right lung, but they couldn't get all the cancerous nodules from the left lung. "He still has tumor problems," Conrad told Greg Kilmer of Nampa's *Idaho Press-Tribune* after the seven-hour operation. "The long-term prognosis is guarded."

Mason was a bit more frank. In the August 20 edition of the *Idaho Statesman*, he was asked by sportswriter Stephen Dodge if he knew what my chances were. "The only thing I know is from talking to his sister," Mason replied. "She asked the doctors for a timeline and they said, 'Well, if he wasn't in such good health we would give him three months, but he's in such good health you never know.'"

But I'm not about to give in. Not after what I have been through. I try not to spend nights worrying about my illness and the bleak odds that face me. I try to enjoy life as best I can while I seek alternative treatments in Canada. I think my career in athletics has instilled in me a perseverance that is going to see me through this. Sure, I've had some tough times, but the sun comes up the next day. And until the sun doesn't come up, I figure I've got a chance.

When you've been in athletics as long as I have, competition becomes part of your life, and I've always enjoyed the role of the underdog. I like to be on the team that is not supposed to win. I used to play a lot of three-on-three basketball, and I'd try to align the players so that my threesome would be outmanned just because I enjoyed the challenge.

This cancer has become the ultimate challenge.

Chapter 16

The Fall of '96

My career is my life. And when my life is at a crossroads, something seems to pull me to Vancouver. When my playing days ended in 1967, I returned to Vancouver. When I got fired by the L.A. Express in 1984, I moved back to Vancouver. When the USFL folded in 1985, I spent a great deal of time in ... well, you get the idea. Beginning with the summer of 1965 western Canada's largest city was my home for most of the next 12 years. When I left in the spring of 1977, Vancouver remained a second home—a haven, a place to be with friends and have some fun and laugh.

Now I'm back. But there's no fun and games this time. I've returned to Vancouver because of my biggest crisis yet: I'm trying to stay alive. It's the fall of 1996 and I'm living in the Vancouver high-rise apartment of my longtime friend Jerry Bradley. I'm here because alternative cancer treatments and experimental drugs—their availability in America hindered by U.S. Food and Drug Administration regulations—are more accessible north of the border. I'm here because I'm told I'm running out of time and conventional Western medicine is not going to cure my affliction. I'm here because I still think I can beat the cancer that has spread to my chest and lungs. But I have to admit, I'm here because I'm running out of options.

Perhaps Paul Buker of the *Oregonian* describes my situation best: "Miracle finishes were a trademark of Allen's teams," he wrote. "Now he needs another one." Buker visited me after I moved in with Bradley following my mid-August cancer surgery in Seattle. "Allen has chased hope to Canada," wrote Buker, whose story appeared in the September 22, 1996, edition of the *Oregonian*. "He's filling himself with experimental drugs, clinging to the hope that something will click—that he will be with his nearly three-year-old daughter, Taylor Elizabeth, next summer in his cabin at Flathead Lake in Montana. That he will simply be alive in six months."

In mid-September a new lump began to grow on my chest. On September 18 I went to Seattle and was told by doctors that my CAT scan results showed that the cancerous lesions had grown. "The doctors seem to think I'm in trouble," I told the *Statesman's* Stephen Dodge around September 19. "And I'm starting to think that I probably am. The cancer cells have not retreated. In fact, they've gotten a little bigger."

Since then, my work on this book consists of talking into a tape recorder; it's the only way I can share my thoughts because my battle with cancer has become a full-time job. These days, I'm up at 6 every weekday morning and on the road in the Ford Explorer borrowed from another long-time friend, Vancouver business owner David Boyd. My destination is Bellingham, Washington, for a 20-minute dose of radiation, designed to shrink the lump in my chest. I know the radiation isn't a cure, but my hope is that the treatment will reduce the tumor enough to buy me some time. By 8:30 the treatment is complete. I hop back in Boyd's vehicle, complete the 110-mile round-trip, and arrive back in Vancouver by 10 a.m. for my appointment at the office of Jim Chan, a naturopathic doctor. For the next six hours I'm in Chan's clinic, hooked up to an intravenous tube that injects hydrogen peroxide, vitamin C and some other drug I can't remember into my system. The idea, Chan says, is to mobilize my white blood cells against the cancer by creating a high-oxygen environment in my bloodstream. I usually get back to Bradley's apartment between 3:45 and 4:30 in the afternoon. I go for an hourlong walk, have a vegetarian dinner and give myself an injection of a medication called 714x. I get the drug from R.H. Rogers, a Vancouver physician who directs the Center for Integrated Therapy in Vancouver. He says 714x contains agents that are supposed to carry nitrogen into the tumors and help my immune system fight the cancerous cells. After dinner I meditate and go to bed—usually by 9.

That's right—meditate. With the help of three cassette tapes, I sit in a reclining position, close my eyes and visualize getting rid of the cancer in my body. The voice on one tape tells me to imagine tiny fish feeding on my cancer cells, gobbling them up like microscopic Pac-Men. I mean, you *know* its desperation time when somebody like me starts meditating.

My daily routine includes drinking a special tea and some other liquid concoctions, which are supposed to fight cancer, and gulping down 80-odd pills a day. And I do mean odd: supplements, herbals, minerals, shark cartilage, human urine crystals, rattlesnake oil. It's all part of what I hope is a cure. I've received all kinds of pills from all kinds of people; I'm willing to try just about anything as long as it isn't toxic. Some of my regular medications can be obtained through physicians in the United States, but since Canada is not regulated by the FDA, the drugs are easier to acquire here in Vancouver.

I've changed my entire lifestyle. Beer and coffee are no longer part of my diet; instead it's carrot juice and porridge. Basically, I'm now a vegetarian, although occasionally I'll have some salmon. Despite what some people believe, I was never a heavy drinker to begin with. Sure, I enjoyed having a few beers, but it wasn't any big deal to give it up; it was just part of the bar scene that I enjoy so much. My new eating habits aren't a huge adjustment; I've always had a pretty healthy diet. I've never eaten a lot of junk food, and I've never been big on sugar or ice cream. Even before I became ill, my diet consisted primarily of chicken, fish and salads.

I hooked up with Dr. Chan through Boyd, who himself was diagnosed with cancer earlier this year, and received treatment from Dr. Rogers with the help of Sherri Niesen, Bradley's ex-girlfriend and another longtime friend of mine who is doing her doctoral work on cancer research at the University of British Columbia. Niesen, the woman who introduced me to my former wife Barbara in 1988, is "a firm believer that meditation, visualization and diet can work wonders," wrote the *Oregonian's* Buker. "She says the mind can both cause and cure disease."

I think Drs. Chan and Rogers have really helped people over the years. But I don't know if they can help someone with rhabdomyosarcoma. I originally thought about going to a clinic in Mexico for more experimental treatment, but I have pretty much ruled that out because it seems no one really seems to know how to deal with this type of cancer when it attacks someone my age. It's a strange disease, vicious and unpredictable. There is nothing this cancer has done that has been normal. When I first got to Vancouver in late August I didn't have the lump in my chest, then it suddenly appeared and started growing like crazy. It was unbelievable how fast it grew. Before I started radiation, I thought the damn thing was going to be bigger than my head. The radiation has since shrunk it considerably, but when you have a lump the size of a fist bulging out of your chest, it's kind of unnerving.

Meanwhile, Bradley and my sister are looking into other possibilities. I'm looking for a cure, but I don't have a clue if the treatment I'm undergoing is helping; I don't think anybody does. My plans could change at any time, but I do know one thing: I'm not going down without a fight. "You either do something, or you die, I guess," I told Buker. "I mean, I don't have a lot of choice, do I? All my choices are bad, but this is the best choice I've got."

My fear isn't so much if I die, but *how* I die. I dread the thought of going out like a whimpering little crybaby. Somebody recently shared with me a saying by a 19th-century writer named Thomas Carlyle: "The courage we desire and prize is not the courage to die decently, but to live manfully." Well, I don't agree. I want to do both. If I die, I want to die a stud. If things don't work out, I want to be remembered as somebody that people respected and who went down with a little class.

I'm handling this situation the only way I know how. I think I'm facing it pretty well because I derive a lot of inner strength from my background in athletics. If my days are numbered, I'm going to make them count. I'm not going to live the remainder of my life whimpering about chemo and being bald and being tired and sick and all these things. I don't plan to simply waste away; I want to live the last days of my life doing things I enjoy—like coaching my team. It's still a goal, a reason to fight on.

The almost unbearable frustration is that I don't feel gravely ill; it's not like I'm in a hospital on a respirator, clinging to life. I could be coaching the Broncos right now. I mean, I could have undergone the surgery in Seattle like I did and still have been back in Boise a week before our August 31 season opener against Central Michigan. After the surgery I could have decided to skip all the alternative treatments, go with just the radiation in Boise once the lump appeared, and coach my ass off the entire fall without a whole lot of problems—I think. But with my current regimen in Vancouver I don't have the time to coach. I did, however, get to see my staff before the '96 opener. Part of the crew flew up to Vancouver the weekend before the CMU game. It was just a little over a week following my surgery, so I was still pretty sore. But I enjoyed seeing them. We talked strategy and barbecued on the balcony at Bradley's apartment. The only thing that was different was my choice of beverage; while most everyone had beer, David Boyd and I sipped cranberry juice and soda.

This whole situation has been quite strange, to say the least. The last time I wasn't actively involved in football was 1956, the year before my freshman season at Missoula County High. It's so god-awful frustrating because after 40 years of playing and coaching, football is what I'm all about. I mean, it's not like I can't discuss strategy and make decisions. But it's awfully damn hard when my team is nearly 700 miles away. "I'm starting to go a little beserko, " I told the *Statesman's* Stephen Dodge two days before our opener, which also marked BSU's first game as a Division I-A team. "I try to stay busy, but mostly I'm just sitting around. I know on Saturday I'm going to be going crazy."

A few weeks later I flew into Boise for a one-day visit to see Carolyn

Collins. I just wanted to slip in and slip out, but I decided to stop by BSU's football offices. When I got there, I was greeted with a lot of good-natured jokes about my healthy appearance. I mean, with the exception of the lump on my chest, I don't look all that sick. "Hey, this medical leave stuff is bullshit," said Barry Sacks with a laugh. "You look fine. Get behind your desk and let's get going!" Believe me, I wanted to.

This cancer is an interesting deal. Here I am fighting for my life, but at the same time I want to coach. The first month in Vancouver wasn't bad because everything was new. But now I'm really itching to return to our program; I'm bored with this treatment stuff. I really miss coaching. I miss my guys—the coaches, the players. I always knew Boise State was a great school to coach for, but now that I'm in exile, so to speak, I really appreciate what a special place it is. BSU has a great atmosphere for college football—maybe as good as anyplace in the West with its blue turf, tailgate parties and enthusiastic crowds. I think the program's potential is limitless. The stadium is outstanding, the school is super, the fan support is second to none, the city is awesome, the weather is great. It's going to take a while to get the program going at the Division I-A level, but Boise is definitely the kind of place where a major college football program can flourish. No question about it.

I haven't been cut off entirely from my team. Since the season began I've kept in touch with interim coach Tom Mason and sports information director Max Corbet on a regular basis. In addition, Corbet sends me video cassettes of our games, and I often talk to him once or twice during our home games while he's in the press box. I have also been able to listen to a few live broadcasts of Bronco home contests by making arrangements with Boise radio station KBOI. Bradley or I will call the station's 800 number and the person at the other end will put us on hold, automatically connecting our phone line to the station's ongoing broadcast—in this case the BSU football game. We'll put the call on the speaker phone and Bradley, Boyd and I will sit back and listen to the play-by-play. That arrangement only works for home games, however, since the station needs its 800 line for its away-game broadcasts. When the Broncos are on the road, we have to pay for the call; it's a good thing Bradley is generous with his money.

Speaking of money, I've been asked how I'm able to pay for these alternative treatments, which aren't covered by insurance. Well, thanks to Bradley and Boyd, my medical costs are just about my only expenses. I've had to empty a couple of bank accounts to pay for the treatments, but I'm living with Bradley for free and I don't have any transportation costs thanks to Boyd, so I've been able to make ends meet that way.

In mid-October I went to a sports bar in downtown Vancouver with Bradley, Boyd and some other friends to watch the BSU-Nevada game from a live satellite hookup. Also in our group was *USA Today* sportswriter Steve Wieberg, who flew to Vancouver to do a story on me. His article accurately captured my frustration as we watched the Broncos get clobbered 66-28: "Mistakes are piling up: an interception, a couple of fumbles, six sacks, a dozen penalties. And Boise State is losing. Big," Wieberg wrote. "Pokey Allen watches the nightmare unfold and shakes his head. 'C'mon,' the Broncos' coach groans. ... But nobody who matters can hear. The players, and the game, are some 700 miles away. Allen is in the back of a sports bar in Vancouver, nursing a bottle of mineral water. He pleads with images on a TV screen.

"What's he doing here, so far removed from the normalcy of his life? Allen wonders himself. He has cancer. Somewhere, he figures, there's a cure. Maybe here, in Canada. Maybe."

IT'S OCTOBER 13, four days before my daughter's third birthday; I still think I can beat this cancer. But it has been a lot harder than I ever imagined. I have my down days, but I still feel pretty good for the most part. So far, this cancer has a tendency to form bumps on my body and not go into organs. And when it does go into my organs, it doesn't grow very fast. One bit of good news is that the lump in my chest has receded, thanks to the radiation. Unfortunately, I recently went to Seattle for a CAT scan and was told the spot on my left lung has grown a little bit, and that worries me. None of the physicians I'm seeing give me much of a chance. But at the same time, none of them will say my situation is irreversible. Carolyn Collins wasn't very optimistic when I went to see her in Boise a few weeks ago, but the one thing she *won't* say is that it's hopeless. Those who are trying to help me aren't going to tell me there's no hope; they won't say that—even if they think it—because if they do and I start to believe them, I'm a goner. If one of my doctors were to say, "Pokey, you've got two months to live," then I'll probably be dead in two months. If a guy with a terminal illness believes that he's going to die in two months, he's usually dead in two months. At this moment, I firmly believe that a fighting attitude and an unyielding determination are my primary weapons in fighting this disease.

One thing I want people to know is that my battle with cancer has not been a solitary ordeal. While the constant uncertainties and often painful and demoralizing side effects of the disease are indeed a personal struggle, I have had incredible support from family and friends every step of the way. My sister and her husband along with friends like Bradley, Boyd and Mike Munsey have been continual sources of help and strength throughout my illness.

With my time-consuming treatments I'm not lacking for things to do, and with Bradley's hospitality and Boyd's companionship I'm definitely not hurting for human contact and support. In fact, isolation and loneliness are the least of my problems these days. I don't mean to be reclusive or unsociable, but I've had to say no to a lot of people who want to come and visit me in Vancouver because I'm either too busy with my treatments during the day or too tired in the evening. I've gone down to Seattle to see Jennie and her family on a couple of occasions, and one weekend my mom and Taylor traveled from Missoula to Seattle so I could meet them there. Spending time with Taylor is both a blessing and a hardship. I love being with her, but it makes me miss her even more when we're apart. I know she's awfully young, but I hope I'm making at least a small impact on her. Whatever happens to me, I hope she realizes that she has a father who really loves her.

BOY, I'M NOT the only one having a bad year. BSU is reeling; after yesterday's loss to Nevada the Broncos' record is 1-6 with two more tough opponents—Utah State and Fresno State—coming up next. I know I've got to make some kind of decision soon in regard to my status at Boise State because I know Gene Bleymaier, the school's athletic director, is in a tough spot. He's got a head coach 700 miles away whose future is in doubt, a team in turmoil, and boosters who have little tolerance for losing—even with our extenuating circumstances. If I can't come back, I would hope that Bleymaier would give the head coaching position to Tom Mason and keep the rest of the coaches. But our record isn't helping matters much. As the season has progressed, my correspondences with Mason and the others have decreased and I've quit watching the videotapes of the games because I realize I can't be of any help. I mean, you can't coach from Vancouver, British Columbia, when your team is in Boise, Idaho. Damn, it's frustrating.

I know it's an awkward situation for everyone back in Boise; I honestly don't know what's going to happen to Mason and the others if I don't make it back. And I'm worried about them. I have a year remaining on my contract after the 1996 season, so everything should be OK if I can return to my post—otherwise, I think the jobs of my assistant coaches may be in jeopardy. That's why I'm still hoping I can find a way to beat this cancer—or at least hold it at bay—in the next two months. To make matters worse, the assistant coaches' contract situation at BSU is a real cause for concern. As head coach, I have a three-year deal, but my assistants have just one-year contracts that run from February 1 to January 31 of each year. Many schools give their assistant football coaches multi-year contracts; at the very least they give them summer-to-summer contracts that allow them some security should they get fired at the end of a season.

I also know my predicament has created a real recruiting problem for Boise State. "Simply put, Allen's situation, and the interim on head coach Tom Mason's title, has become a stone anchor to this staff," wrote the *Statesman's* Stephen Dodge in early October. In Dodge's article, Mason said he knew for a fact that Idaho, Utah State and UNLV were using our program's unstable situation due to my illness against us in the recruiting wars. "It's the nature of the business," Mason said. "Most coaches, if they are any good, have every article on Pokey laminated and in their briefcase."

I can't argue with Dodge's assessment, but I do blame his employer for part of our problem. Certainly, it's not the *Statesman's* job to recruit BSU football players, but all the negative publicity we received in the paper the previous year has provided other programs with abundant ammunition to scare away potential recruits. For example, Utah State laminated several negative *Statesman* stories about our program that were printed in 1995. So, as Mason asserts, when a USU recruiter goes into the home of a player, he can pull out the articles and say something like, "Hey, look at this. Look at what the local newspaper in Boise does to the BSU football program. The paper crucified the quarterback. It put mug shots of 17 players in the paper. Do you want to put up with that kind of shit there?"

To be sure, recruiting is a competitive part of the coaching business, and I know the local newspaper is not supposed to be a mouthpiece for the local college, but there is no question that the *Statesman's* excessive coverage of our team's problems in 1995 is still hurting the program in 1996.

As mentioned earlier, another reason for BSU's current woes is the backlash from our quick fix with junior college transfers following our disastrous first season. After we went 3-8 in 1993 I knew we needed to turn things around posthaste with an infusion of JC imports. "It worked in the short term as Allen's Broncos went to the I-AA national championship game in 1994," the *Statesman's* Dodge noted earlier this month, "but it's hurting the team now." No kidding. With the outstanding junior college crop we recruited after the 1993 season, our staff had high hopes for banner years in both '94 and '95. But with our off-the-field problems and my illness in 1995, we seemed to lack focus and enthusiasm and failed to recapture the magic of '94 despite the fact our starting lineup was filled with seniors—both JC imports and non-transfers—from the previous year's national runner-up squad. And the situation is much tougher this year with our entry into Division I-A football.

Our emphasis on signing JC players two and a half years ago combined with the current constraints in reaching the Division I-A scholarship level of 85 has left our team with a huge void in experienced players. Basically, we graduated something like 24 seniors after the 1995 season and replaced them with 24 freshmen. Tom Mason has had no choice but to pull true freshmen off the redshirt list and insert them in the lineup. I mean, a year ago some of these kids were playing high school football and now they're going up against the likes of Arizona State. Sure, it's all part of becoming a big-time program. My only point is that people need to realize that this situation was unavoidable. "BSU," wrote Dodge, "is paying for the quick fix right now."

Boy, are we ever. A lack of luck, depth and experience has just killed us so far this year. When Mason and the other coaches came to visit me in Vancouver in August, I remember sitting out on Jerry Bradley's balcony and telling them this season was going to be a struggle—a major struggle. "With the possible exception of Portland State, we are not better than anybody we're going to play this year," I said. "The only thing we have better than most of our opponents is an experienced senior quarterback in Tony Hilde. That's it. That is our only plus. And one player is not going to make that much difference."

Still, I didn't expect our first season as a Division I-A team to be *this* tough.

IN LATE OCTOBER I had my final radiation treatment. A week or so later, the tumor in my chest unexpectedly burst; in a matter of days it shrank noticeably. For several days fluid oozed from the tumor, leaking through the bandages on my chest and staining my shirts. It was messy, but I started feeling better. Soon after, I had a CAT scan that didn't detect any active cancer cells in what remained of the tumor. Furthermore, the cancerous cells in my lung, although alive, were growing at a very slow rate and were causing me no problems. A few days later, during the first week of November, I started feeling stronger almost overnight as the lump in my chest continued to shrink. "Hey," I thought, "this tumor is getting smaller and I'm feeling better. Maybe I can coach again."

I wasn't fooling myself—or anyone else. I knew I wasn't cured. But the ruptured tumor in my chest and stagnant cancer cells in my lungs were what I was hoping for—the kind of breakthrough that I thought could allow me to return to Boise and my football team. On Friday, November 8, I continued to feel better and considered myself healthy enough to return to the rigors of my job at BSU; I wasted no time. That morning I called Tom Mason and Gene Bleymaier. "I want to come back," I said. "What do you think?" Neither one hesitated. "Hey, come on back," Mason responded. "Your office is still open." That's all it took; I was going to return to Boise. The next day BSU lost to North Texas 30-27 on a last-second field goal to fall to 1-9. It was our eighth straight loss and one of the lowest points in the history of football at BSU. The next night, Sunday, November 10, I flew to Boise. BSU had two games remaining—on the road at New Mexico State and at home against Idaho.

I've never been one to wax philosophical, so I'm not going to do it now in explaining why I returned to the BSU football program on November 11. It was just something I had to do. I was tired of the treatments. I was tired of going from doctor to doctor looking for a cure. I don't know how or why my condition improved, but it did. And from what I've been told, a tumor—even one that's been blasted with radiation—doesn't usually liquify and burst like mine did, but it did. There was no reason for me to come back unless my health improved, and it did. I mean, I couldn't coach with that tumor sticking out of my chest. But after it burst, well, that allowed me to contemplate a return.

I probably would not have rejoined the team if we had been 5-5 or had a winning record. But given the circumstances, I thought I could help Tom Mason and the rest of our staff. Like I said, my decision to return had been made before the North Texas game and with Bleymaier's and Mason's consent; the outcome of that contest had no bearing on my decision. I simply wanted to return to the job I love and inject some life into our program for our two remaining games. "If I didn't think I'd have a positive effect, I'd stay up here the next two months," I told the *Statesman's* Mike Prater in a telephone interview before I headed to the Vancouver airport to fly to Boise.

Media reports said I wanted to get Carolyn Collins' OK the morning of November 11 before I officially rejoined the program that afternoon. But I had already made up my mind: I was going to coach. All I wanted her to do was confirm that the cancer wasn't behaving aggressively and that I didn't have anything seriously wrong. My only physical problem was some soreness and muscle spasms in my neck and shoulders. I attributed that pain to the radiation and the fact that the muscles and skin in that area had previously been stretched by the tumor and were now readjusting to their natural alignment.

When asked about my recovery, Collins seemed to be as surprised as anyone. "For the moment, he is stable and for whatever reason that is true," she told the *Statesman*. "Whatever caused that I'm quite grateful." Collins told the paper that she expected the malignant nodules in my lungs to have "doubled, tripled or even quadrupled in size by now." Instead, she said, they are the same size as when I left BSU on August 6.

November 11 was a whirlwind. After meeting with Collins I attended the noon luncheon of the Bronco Athletic Association for my first public appearance in Boise since the August 6 press conference when I announced I was stepping down. Chris Bouneff of the *Idaho Press-Tribune* described me as a "grayer and gaunter" version of the person who left Boise in August. Well, maybe I didn't look so good, but being back at BSU was the best prescription imaginable. Still, I knew I had to convince the skeptics that my return wasn't some last hurrah—not just a two-game stint before my time was up.

"I didn't come back just to coach two games," I told the capacity crowd in the BSU Student Union. "I wouldn't do that to the people of Boise. I wouldn't come back for a short-term arrangement. Being in Boise and coaching this football team and being around you people is the best medicine I could have. I didn't come back like I did a year ago when I was gonna nap all day—I'm not napping—I'm back to coach. If it takes 16 to 18 hours, that's what I'll do. I'll work 16 to 18 hours and sleep for six if that is what it takes. You're getting a full-timer here. I think there is always the chance of the cancer coming back with anybody. But I think right now that I'm in great shape. I've got a great chance of not having anything bad happen for the next three or four years, at least."

I'm not an emotional person, but I also tried to convey my feelings to the crowd— to tell my friends and supporters how important it was for me to be back. "The one thing that I didn't realize when I went to Canada is how much I'd miss Boise and Boise State and you people," I said. "This is the best place there is, and we're going to get it done. This program is going to be one of the top football programs in the country in the next one and a half to two years. I'm not promising anything because I think Tom Mason is as talented a coach as there is. I hope I can add a little inspiration to this football team and I hope we can win the next two games. I've been coaching 29 years now and I've been in this position before. It's a hard thing once you start losing—especially with a young team—to turn that around. But I hope we can turn it around—not just for this year, but for next year."

That afternoon—amid much media hoopla—I was back with my team. But before we hit the practice field, my first order of business was to hold a closed-door meeting with my players and coaches. Earlier in the season I had spoken briefly to the players when I made my one-day visit to Boise. But this time I had plenty to say. It wasn't an emotional gathering, at least from my perspective. My purpose was to reiterate what I had said at the BAA luncheon. I wanted to assure everyone that I wasn't back for just two games. I told them I had returned because my health had improved and I thought I could help. But my main message was aimed at the players: This losing is unacceptable, I told them, and it won't continue.

I wasn't sure what kind of emotional impact, if any, my return would have on our team; neither did anyone else. "Whether this latest twist translates into victories, no one is certain," observed the *Statesman's* Prater. Sure, I was trying to rally the troops and salvage something from an abysmal season. But you still need the talent to win, and none of us were sure we had the horses to beat New Mexico State, even though the Aggies were going through an equally wretched season. Said Mason, "I don't know if we're good enough to rally and win one for the Gipper."

BOISE STATE VS. New Mexico State. Let's face it, our identical records said it all: 1-9. Everyone knew our contest with the Aggies pitted two football programs in disarray. At the same time that I was returning to BSU, NMSU head coach Jim Hess announced that he was stepping down following our November 16 contest, the Aggies' season finale. Had it not been for the intrigue surrounding my return and Hess' impending departure, our game in Las Cruces would have been the yawner of the year. Still, our coaching staff worked long, hard hours that week, trying to find a way to end our eight-game losing streak.

And a few days later, in 43 remarkable seconds on a wind-whipped football field in the high desert of the Southwest, I knew why I fought so hard to come back and coach.

As the *Idaho Statesman's* headline blared the next morning, it was "Unbelievable!" In an improbable comeback made more dramatic by my return to the sidelines, we edged New Mexico State 33-32. "A minute earlier the Broncos were certain losers," wrote the *Statesman's* Dodge. "New Mexico State had driven 80 yards for the go-ahead touchdown with 43 seconds remaining. The Broncos were finished, defeated, just like every other Saturday in the team's dismal, school-record eight-game losing streak. ... But a funny thing happened on the way to humiliation. Ryan Ikebe picked up a bobbled kickoff return and handed it to Andre Horace on a reverse. Horace turned the corner and found daylight … and was finally tackled on the New Mexico State 22-yard line."

We had no timeouts with 27 seconds remaining. Hilde, who had suffered a broken rib earlier in the game, threw an incomplete pass to Ikebe in the end zone. Twenty seconds remained. Offensive coordinator Dave Stromswold called the same play to the other side of the field. "Hilde hung in the pocket and released the ball just as he was drilled by a blitzing Aggie," Dodge wrote. "The pass fluttered. Ikebe turned at the last moment, spun toward the inside, and fell into the end zone with Hilde's pass cradled safely to his chest. Touchdown. Broncos win. Insanity reigned."

It was a wild, incredible scene on the sidelines. "The players yelled," Dodge said. "They mobbed one another. Some even cried, overcome with emotion when the Broncos snatched victory away from another certain defeat." Sure, I was excited about emerging victorious in my debut as a Division I-A coach and helping BSU gain its first victory in the Big West Conference—but I was more excited about simply being on the sidelines, coaching again. I mean, you can't put too much stock in one victory against a mediocre opponent at the end of an awful season.

I think Dodge put the game in the right perspective: "This wasn't about football. It concerned Pokey Allen, a man the players loved. Many believed they'd never see him on the field again—and yet there he was, a magician pulling victory from his sleeves, inspiring the end of an eight-game losing streak."

Given all I had been through and how I had fought back, I think people wanted me to gush about how emotionally overwhelmed I was by it all. Sure it was emotional, but I'm not the type to wear my feelings on my sleeve. Truth is, I was exhausted and I was disappointed because we didn't play well, especially on defense. Given the numbers our defense yielded to NMSU, we should have lost. To be brutally honest, two bad teams met that day, and one of them had to win. Luckily, it was us.

The euphoria of our victory in Las Cruces ended with a resounding thud the following Saturday as we got hammered by Idaho 64-19 in our season finale. We needed more than luck to beat the Vandals; we were overmatched at virtually every position and it showed. What happened was predictable, but I don't think that matters with our boosters. And I don't think our staff is going to get too many more chances to beat Idaho again.

IT'S FRIDAY, NOVEMBER 29, the day after Thanksgiving 1996. I'm sitting in the living room of the town house I share with BSU wrestling coach Mike Young. I just finished watching the nationally televised special segment that CBS Sports did on my return to the Boise State football program. My comeback from my sickbed has attracted considerable media attention. It's been chronicled in *Sports Illustrated* and several other publications. It's been described as "great theater," "Hollywood material" and "the stuff of storybooks." That's all very nice, but these last 23 months have been anything but a fairy tale. I'm not particularly interested in personal publicity and glory. I came back simply because I wanted to do the job I was hired to do.

What are my future plans now that the 1996 season is over? I assume we're going to have a great recruiting year because our staff has always had one when we've been put in a rebuilding position. I assume we're going to have great spring practices and a great conditioning program, and I think we're going to have a good football team come next fall. Like I said when I first returned, I'm here for the duration. "Stagnant," "inactive" and "under control" are the words used most often to describe the malignancies in my body right now. And that's fine. I'm ready to roll.

Right now I feel good. I don't have any problems. I continue to take dozens of pills and other concoctions and maintain my strictly vegetarian diet. I haven't had a CAT scan for about three weeks, but as far as I know, I don't have any cancer cells that are overly active. Except for my stiff neck and my shoulder problem, I feel good. I've been asked what happens if the cancer returns. Well, it's simple: I'm gone and I'm not coming back to coach at BSU. I don't know what contingency plans Gene Bleymaier has, but I don't really care because I don't think I'm going to get sick again.

Chapter 17

Fourth and Long

Cancer is a wicked and virulent enemy, unleashing its destruction on the best of us. On the afternoon of December 11 on the Boise State campus there were two sad reminders of its terrible power.

First was the university's memorial service honoring Larry Selland, BSU's former executive vice president, who died of cancer in his Boise home a few days earlier. Second was the announcement that I was resigning the head coaching position effective immediately because a CAT scan revealed that the cancer cells in my lungs were once again active.

The CAT scan was taken at the St. Alphonsus Cancer Treatment Center on December 10. My sister Jennie was in Boise at the time, so she went with me to have the CAT scan taken and get the results from Dr. Carolyn Collins, my oncologist. When we met with Collins to get her prognosis, I could tell something was wrong by the look on her face.

"Pokey, the news is bad," Collins said. "Real bad. There's been a lot of change in your lungs. The disease has spread, and I'm certain that it's going to continue to grow."

I looked over at my sister, and she started crying; I just sat there, shocked. The news was really hard to take because I had two great CAT scans in a row before this one, and those results gave me a lot of hope that the cancer was still under control. "Well," I said to Collins, "what do we do now?"

But I already knew the answer.

Jennie and I talked a little bit after Dr. Collins gave me the bad news. "I have to resign," I said. "I have no choice. I need to head back to Vancouver." The alternative treatments I received in Canada seemed to slow the cancer's growth, and I'm hoping it can happen again.

At 10 a.m. December 11, I told my staff I was stepping down. After

the 2 p.m. memorial service for Larry Selland, Max Corbet, our sports information director, sent out the news release.

IT'S MONDAY AFTERNOON, December 16. I'm in my office in the Boise
State Varsity Center. Patti Morgan, the football program's office coordinator, is helping me clear out—emptying bookshelves and drawers, remov-
ing pictures from the walls, filling boxes—as I sit at my desk.

Tomorrow is the second anniversary of BSU's appearance in the Division I-AA national championship game. A helluva lot has happened to
me since then. Also tomorrow my friend Bubby Cronin, a Portland businessman, is going to fly to Boise and take me back to Vancouver in his
private plane.

There has been a steady stream of well-wishers—friends, boosters,
my assistant coaches—coming by throughout the day. There are a lot of
red and puffy eyes. I don't feel real good, physically and emotionally, right
now. I'm hurt and disappointed because I couldn't come back all the way
and because I won't coach at BSU anymore. I came back trying to have it
all—my job, my health, living in Boise—and I guess I shouldn't have come
back. I'm not going to get it all, so I might as well decide just to concentrate on trying to beat cancer and not worry about anything else for right
now. I have cancer cells covering my lungs. If it continues the way it's going, I might only have a month to live. There's nothing that I'm doing in
Boise that is going to eradicate the cancer in my lungs, so I've got to go
somewhere where at least I've got a chance. I'm not quitting. I'm going to
fight this disease. I want to beat it and I want to coach again—and to do
that I had to resign.

I plan to return to Jerry Bradley's apartment, get situated there, and
weigh my options. Right now I plan to see Jim Chan and R.H. Rogers, the
two Vancouver doctors who provided me with my alternative cancer treatments this fall. I'll discuss my alternatives with them and go from there;
I'll return to the six hours of IVs in Chan's clinic and the rest of the routine I was following in Vancouver if I have to. I'm also going to Missoula
for Christmas. After all, I have to see my daughter, Taylor, and my mom,
and I have plans to be with Mike Munsey at The Depot Christmas Eve.
Tradition, you know.

I guess I could rage at the injustice and unfairness of it all. I want to
see my daughter grow up. But if I die, I know she's going to be fine. She
has a good mom and she's going to have a good life. But like I said almost
two years ago, Why *not* me?

I thought I was going to beat it. But now I don't know. I'm disappointed and unhappy, but I don't have any real heavy emotions. I want to live, but I'm not afraid to die. Maybe I will be afraid when I'm lying in a hospital bed and the end is near. But I've never been afraid to die.